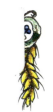

Spice of Life SPECIALTY FOODS
PRESENTS
Common Sense Cooking

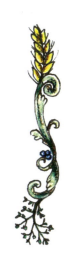

Edith Maki

*all the best.
Edith Maki*

Spice of Life Specialty Foods, LLC
Hancock, Michigan

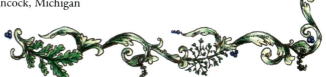

Spice of Life Specialty Foods Presents Common Sense Cooking.
Copyright 2012 © 2013 by Edith Maki. All rights reserved. Published by Spice of Life Specialty Foods, LLC. Printed in the United States of America by Book Concern Printers in Hancock, Michigan. No part of this book may be used or reproduced in any manner whatsoever without written permission except in the case of brief quotations embodied in critical articles and reviews and as provided by USA copyright law.

Written/edited by Edith Maki. Photographs by Eevi Maki and Edith Maki.
Illustration/design by Eevi Maki.

Second Edition

ISBN: 978-0-9885699-1-1

Contents

Notes: v
Trocomare®: v
Celery: v
Eggs: v
Baking/Cooking Temperatures v
Yeast v
Baking Powder v
Spice Chart vi
Foreward ix
Gluten-Free Helps & Hints x

PICKLES & PRESERVES

Bread and Butter Pickles 1
Olive Oil Pickles 2
Dill Pickles 3
Counter Top Dill Pickles 4
Celery Chow Chow 5
Pickled Beets 6
Sauerkraut 7
Basic Tomato Sauce 8
Victoria's Salsa 9
Whole Cranberry Sauce 10
Berry Sauce: for waffles, etc. 11
Low/Alternate Sugar Jam or Jelly 12
Wild Blackberry Jelly 13
Currant Jelly 13
Pepperidge Farm Style Apricot Jam 14

SIDE DISHES

Fluffy Millet Side Dish 15
Buckwheat Kasha 16
Bread Stuffing 17
Rice Stuffing 18
Allspiced Cider 19
Nori Rolls (Sushi) 20
Savory Scalloped Potatoes 21

Common Sense Cooking

SOUPS

Chicken Vegetable Soup 22
Chicken Noodle Soup 23
Heart Warming Turkey Soup 24
Split Pea Soup 25
Basic Miso Soup 26
Hunter's Stew 27
Beef Chili 28
Baked Beans 29

SALADS

Basic Blender Mayonnaise 30
Italian Style Salad Dressing...31
Homemade Blue Cheese Salad Dressing........................31
Elsie's Cream Cheese Salad Dressing..............................32
French Garden Salad (Salade Niçoise) 33
Traditional Cole Slaw 34
Zucchini Dulse Salad 35
Wild Rice Salad..36
Rice Garbanzo Salad...37
Potato Salad 38
Tuna Noodle Salad 39
Mixed Bean Salad 40
Three Bean Salad 41
Beet-Herring Salad (Rosolli)..42
Cranberry Ring Salad 43

SANDWICH SPREADS

Pam's Pepper Cheese Spread 44
Chicken Salad Spread 45
Tuna Salad Spread 46
Egg Salad Spread 47
Hummus...48

GLUTEN FREE

Gluten-Free Pulla (Nisu) 114
Gluten-Free Gingerbread..115

Spice of Life Specialty Foods PRESENTS

BREADS

- Granola 49
- Cinnamon Granola 49
- Limppu Rye Bread 50
- Finnish Sourdough Rye Bread 51
- Wheat Bread 52
- Multigrain Bread 53
- Whole Wheat Yeast Waffles 54
- Whole Wheat Pancakes 55
- Whole Wheat Blueberry Muffins 56
- Zucchini Bread 57
- Finnish Cardamom Bread/Pulla/Nisu 58
- Cinnamon Buns 59
- Fruit & Nut Filled Buns: 60
- Cinnamon Rolls 61

MAIN DISHES

- Spaghetti 62
- Turkey Rice Casserole 63
- Marinade for Lamb Roast 64
- Marinade for Grilled Turkey 65
- Grilled Whole Turkey 66
- Basting Sauce or Marinade for Grilled Fish or Chicken 67
- Grilled Chicken Marinades 68
- Lemon Herb Marinade 68
- Teriyaki Marinade 69
- Spicy Marinade 69
- Baked Fish Fillets in Tomato Sauce 70
- Potato Pancakes 71
- Seafood Lasagna 72
- Lasagna 73
- Fried Fish 74
- Lamb or Beef Meatballs 75
- Turkey Meatballs 76
- Mushroom Sauce 77
- Finnish Karelian Pastries/Karjalan Piirakkas 78
- Pasty 80
- Pizza from Scratch 81

Common Sense Cooking

CAKES & PIES

Rhubarb Custard Pie 82
Baked Cheesecake 83
No-Bake Strawberry Cheesecake 84
Raspberry-Filled Cake 85
Raspberry Cream Pie 86
Raspberry Sauce 87
Carrot Cake 88
Our Favorite Fruit Cake 89
Pie Crust 90
Gluten-Free Pie Crust 90
Pumpkin Pie 91
Bavarian Cream Pie 92
Grandma's Blueberry Pie Filling 93
Zucchini Pie 94
Rose Hip Sauce 95
Zucchini Lemon Sauce 96
Zucchini Gingerbread 97

COOKIES & BARS

Chocolate Chip Cookies 98
Cranberry White Chocolate Chip Cookies 99
Finnish Cardamom Cookies 100
Cardamom White Caps 101
Ginger Snaps 102
Finnish Ginger Cookies 103
Pumpkin Cookies 104
German Peppernuts 105
Macaroons 106
Pecan Tarts 107
Granola Chews 108
Chocolate Caramel Bars 109
Blueberry Bars 110
Apple Pastry 111
Chocolate Truffle 112
Caramel Corn 113

Index 116

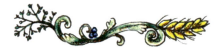

Spice of Life Specialty Foods PRESENTS

NOTES:

Baking/Cooking Temperatures:
We have found that every stove cooks slightly different: gas, electric, old, new, etc. You'll need to try your stove. When baking, check item half-way through as well as ten minutes before time required. Your stove may require you to cook items longer. You also need to consider how high you live above sea level. We found this makes a difference in some items—adjust recipe accordingly.

Baking Powder:
If you have health concerns about the aluminum in baking powder, we recommend that you use Rumford® Aluminum-Free baking powder for any recipes that call for baking powder. This is the brand we use in these recipes. If you find another aluminum-free brand, that should work as well.

Cardamom:
Freshly ground cardamom has the best flavor for baking. However, if you only have access to pre-ground cardamom, that will work also. You will want to double the quantity for better flavor.

Celery:
The outer few stalks of celery are usually tougher and are better to be used in soups or other cooked or fried recipes. For recipes that use celery raw, use stalks from an inner layer.

Eggs:
When a recipe calls for separating eggs, it's important to follow those directions. If you end up with extra egg white, use them for macaroons or meringues. If you end up with extra egg yolk, make a custard or pudding.

Yeast:
Active dry yeast is listed in some recipes. SAF is an instant yeast that can be used also and goes in anytime except in extremely hot water. A few other brands of instant yeast are Red Star and Fleischmans.

Salad Oil:
Salad oil is often a mix of other oils. These oils can be mixed in any proportions. Extra-Virgin olive oil is often not as noticeable when mixed with other oils. Oils to use are: olive, almond, walnut, rice bran, and grapeseed.

Trocomare®:
A. Vogel's Trocomare® is an organic spicy herb seasoning salt that we found to be a great source of added flavor without MSG. We have found it at the local co-op, but you could try a health food store, the healthy section of the grocery store, check online, or make a special request at a store. The reason for the flavor is the ingredients: Sea salt, organic vegetables and herbs (organic celery, organic leek, organic cress, organic onion, organic chives, organic parsley, organic lovage, organic red pepper, organic garlic, organic horseradish, organic basil, organic marjoram, organic rosemary, organic thyme), kelp (with trace iodine). Most other seasoned salts do not compare to this flavor. The company that distributes this is:
Hershey Import Co.
96 Executive Avenue
Edison, NJ 08817 USA
If you're interested, a milder version of this is called Herbamare®.

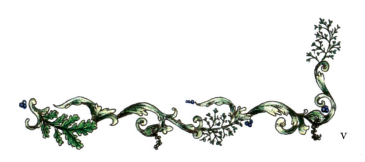

Common Sense Cooking

Spice Chart

Feel free to use herbs and spices, and use what you have whether fresh or dried. Herbs and spices add to the flavor of food. Start by using a couple flavors in a dish in order to learn to distinguish flavors and recognize which ones go together. Add more as you gain confidence.

Soups

All soups: onion, celery, and pepper
Bean soup: bay leaf, basil, savory, thyme, mustard, dash of cloves
Chicken soup: nutmeg, rosemary, marjoram, dill seed
Chowder: poultry seasoning, oregano, thyme
Cream soup (chicken or potato): mace, paprika
Cream soup (tomato and pea): cloves, paprika, basil, oregano
Oyster stew: dash of mace, liberal amount of paprika, marjoram
Potato soup: rosemary, sage, dill seed, basil
Split pea soup: thyme, bay leaf, dash of nutmeg, rosemary, mint
Lentil soup: savory
Vegetable soup: thyme, garlic, basil, mustard seed

Fish and Shellfish

Any baked or broiled fish: bay leaf, onion powder, dill, marjoram, thyme, savory, basil
Poached fish: rosemary, thyme
Shrimp: basil, oregano, rosemary, thyme
Tuna: basil, thyme
Seafood cocktails and spreads: basil, thyme, cayenne, parsley

Meats

Roast beef: onion, garlic
Pot roast: cloves, allspice, bay leaf, ginger, onion, garlic
Beef stew: onion, celery, bay leaf, rosemary, dash of nutmeg
Meat loaf: celery, onion, cloves or allspice, dill seed
Liver: basil, thyme, sage, oregano, onion, garlic, marjoram
Pork: sage, allspice, basil, thyme, rosemary, ginger, celery
Ham: whole cloves, mustard
Veal: onion, celery, poultry seasoning, curry, rosemary
Lamb: curry, basil, oregano, sage, thyme, rosemary, celery, mint
Venison: onions, basil, thyme
Poultry and stuffings: onion, celery, garlic, paprika, basil, oregano, sage, thyme, rosemary, marjoram, savory, parsley flakes

Salads and dressings

Avocado: onion, chili powder, oregano
Cole slaw: paprika, thyme, dill seed, marjoram
Cottage cheese: onion, sage, thyme, marjoram, caraway or dill seed
Fruit: basil, rosemary or mint
Mixed green: basil, oregano, savory, marjoram
Potato: green onion, celery, oregano, caraway, dill seed, savory, marjoram
Seafood: basil, oregano
Cooked salad dressing: pepper, mustard, paprika
French dressing: dash of curry
Tomato aspic: thyme

Spice of Life Specialty Foods PRESENTS

Vegetables
Asparagus: thyme, basil, savory, marjoram
Baked beans: mustard, ginger, bit of allspice
Broccoli: oregano, marjoram
Cabbage: onion, celery, thyme, oregano, sage, basil, savory, marjoram, curry, caraway seed
Carrots: sage, thyme, basil, ginger, dill, marjoram
Cauliflower: rosemary, dill
Corn: dash of chili powder, paprika
Cucumber: rosemary, basil, marjoram, thyme, savory
Eggplant or summer squash: allspice, bay leaf, sage, basil, garlic, green pepper, onion, thyme, oregano, rosemary, savory, marjoram
Lima beans: celery, onion, sage, savory, basil, marjoram
Mushrooms: oregano, savory, onion, garlic, paprika, marjoram
Onion: basil, oregano, sage, thyme
Peas: basil, sage, rosemary, thyme, marjoram, dill or mint
Baked potato: paprika, chives, dill, marjoram
Boiled potato: caraway seed, parsley flakes, chives
Sauerkraut: caraway seed, dill seed
Spinach: dash of nutmeg, rosemary, thyme, oregano
Squash: cinnamon
String beans: basil, garlic, celery salt, thyme, marjoram
Sweet potatoes: dash of nutmeg, cloves
Swiss chard: onion
Tomatoes: allspice, basil, bay leaf, oregano, rosemary, savory, thyme, marjoram

Cheese
Welsh rarebit or fondue: basil, paprika, mustard, oregano, marjoram
Souffles: basil, oregano, sage, thyme, rosemary
Cream cheese spread: onion, garlic, oregano, thyme, dill, hot peppers, caraway seed
Dips: onion, garlic, parsley, dill

Eggs
Scrambled or omelets: basil, oregano, thyme, rosemary, cayenne, tabasco sauce, marjoram
Deviled or egg salad: thyme, rosemary, cayenne, sage, marjoram

Coffee breads, rolls, biscuits
Biscuits: onion, grated cheese added to dough
Coffee cake: cinnamon topping
Doughnuts: dash of mace in batter, nutmeg, anise
Muffins: touch of cinnamon, or nutmeg to enhance flavor
Bread rolls: sprinkle with poppy seed or sesame

Puddings, pies and cakes
Apple: cinnamon and/or nutmeg
Cherry: dash of mace
Chocolate: cinnamon or mace
Custard: nutmeg
Mince: allspice, cinnamon, cloves
Peach: sprinkle of cinnamon, ginger
Pumpkin: cinnamon, cloves, nutmeg, ginger
Raisin: cinnamon
Rhubarb: nutmeg
Rice pudding: cinnamon, nutmeg

Foreword

In the late 1950's, before I was 10 years old I moved with my family from the big city of Minneapolis to a farm in the country. My parents went "back to the earth" years before it was "hip". On the farm we grew our own vegetables and raised chickens and beef for meat, milk and eggs. We ground our own wheat for flour to bake whole wheat bread at the advice of Adele Davis and J.I. Rodale, the pioneers in nutritional awareness. As a member of a large family I had no lack of opportunities to cook and bake. I developed my culinary skills cooking from scratch and making "health foods". After high school graduation, I spent a year living in Finland as a kotiapulainen (home-helper). Besides taking care of children, it was my duty to cook some of the meals. It was there I made my acquaintance with authentic Finnish foods. When I became a wife and mother I brought along various recipes that had developed through those years. They got further testing in our home kitchen on our children and friends. In the early 1990's I was asked to write a cooking column for our local newspaper. For almost three years in *Common Sense Cooking*, I shared nutritional concepts as well as recipes for cooking, baking, canning, and preserving. In 2003, I had the opportunity to operate a deli/bakery, Spice of Life Specialty Foods, where the items we offered our customers were made using some of our favorite recipes. This book contains a selection of those — ENJOY!

— *Edith Maki*

GLUTEN-FREE HINTS AND HELPS:

Gluten-free recipes:
Apricot Jam, Pepperidge Farm Style .. 14
Allspiced Cider.................................. 19
Baked Beans..................................... 29
Bean Salad................................. 40, 41
Beef Chili... 28
Beet-Herring Salad (Rosolli).............. 42
Berry Sauce: for waffles, etc. 11
Blackberry Jelly 13
Blue Cheese Dressing 31
Bread and Butter Pickles..................... 1
Buckwheat Kasha 16
Caramel Corn 113
Chicken Salad Spread 45
Chicken Vegetable Soup 22
Cole Slaw 34
Cranberry Ring Salad 43
Cranberry Sauce 10
Cream Cheese Salad Dressing........... 32
Currant Jelly..................................... 13
Dill Pickles... 3
Dill Pickles, Counter Top 4
Egg Salad Spread 47
Fluffy Millet Side Dish 15
French Garden Salad (Salade Niçoise) 33
Grandma's Blueberry Pie Filling 93
Gluten-Free Gingerbread................. 115
Gluten-Free Pie Crust 90
Gluten-Free Pulla (Nisu) 114
Hunter's Stew (with potatoes)........... 27
Italian Style Salad Dressing............... 31
Jam or Jelly, Low/Alternate Sugar 12
Lemon Herb Marinade..................... 68
Macaroons...................................... 106
Marinade for Grilled Fish/Chicken.... 67
Mayonnaise...................................... 30
Nori Rolls (Sushi).............................. 20
Olive Oil Pickles 2
Pam's Pepper Cheese Spread 44
Pickled Beets 6
Potato Pancakes 71
Potato Salad 38
Pumpkin Pie (filling)........................ 91
Raspberry Sauce 87
Rice Garbanzo Salad......................... 37
Rose Hip Sauce 95
Sauerkraut... 7
Tomato Sauce..................................... 8
Tuna Salad Spread 46
Turkey Rice Casserole....................... 63
Turkey Soup 24
Victoria's Salsa 9
Wild Rice Salad 36
Zucchini Dulse Salad 35
Zucchini Lemon Sauce 96

Recipes to substitute gluten-free pasta:
Chicken Noodle Soup 23
Lasagna 73
Seafood Lasagna 72
Spaghetti 62
Tuna Noodle Salad 39

Recipes to substitute gluten-free flour:
Apple Pastry 111
Baked Fish Fillets in Tomato Sauce.... 70
Blueberry Bars 110
Cardamom White Caps................... 101
Carrot Cake 88
Celery Chow Chow............................. 5
Chocolate Caramel Bars 109
Chocolate Chip Cookies 98
Cranberry White Chocolate Chip
Cookies 99
Finnish Cardamom Cookies............ 100
Finnish Ginger Cookies................... 103
German Peppernuts........................ 105
Ginger Snaps 102
Granola Chews............................... 108
Lamb or Beef Meatballs.................... 75
No-Bake Strawberry Cheesecake 84
Our Favorite Fruit Cake 89
Pasty... 80
Pecan Tarts 107
Pie Crust 90
Pizza from Scratch 81
Pumpkin Cookies........................... 104
Raspberry-Filled Cake 85
Rhubarb Custard Pie 82
Savory Scalloped Potatoes................ 21
Turkey Meatballs 76
Zucchini Gingerbread 97
Zucchini Pie..................................... 94

Recipes to substitute gluten-free cookies:
Baked Cheesecake 83
Bavarian Cream Pie 92
Raspberry Cream Pie........................ 86

Recipes to substitute gluten-free bread:
Bread Stuffing 17
Rice Stuffing..................................... 18

Recipe to substitute gluten-free crackers and bread:
Fried Fish 74

Recipes to make sure to use brown rice miso (no gluten in it):
Basic Miso Soup 26
Hummus.. 48
Split Pea Soup 25

Recipes to make sure to use tamari (usually gluten-free) or gluten-free soy sauce:
Marinade for Grilled Turkey............. 65
Marinade for Lamb Roast................. 64
Mushroom Sauce.............................. 77
Spicy Marinade 69
Teriyaki Marinade 69

Recipes to substitute gluten-free oats:
Cinnamon Granola 49
Granola 49

Recipes to substitute pure chocolate:
Chocolate Truffle............................ 112

Make sure to purchase pure chocolate for your baking so that it's gluten-free.

There are many Web sites that offer gluten-free advice, information, and baking tips, but no advice is so helpful as baking and testing recipes yourself.

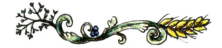

Spice of Life Specialty Foods PRESENTS

Bread and Butter Pickles

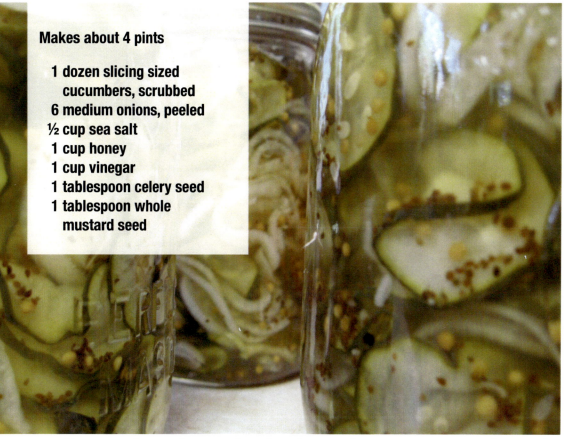

Makes about 4 pints

- 1 dozen slicing sized cucumbers, scrubbed
- 6 medium onions, peeled
- ½ cup sea salt
- 1 cup honey
- 1 cup vinegar
- 1 tablespoon celery seed
- 1 tablespoon whole mustard seed

Slice cucumbers and onions thin. Dissolve sea salt in 2 quarts water. Soak cucumbers and onion slices in the salt water overnight. The next morning, drain well. Scrub and sterilize 4 pint jars with lids and rings. In a large kettle, boil honey and vinegar with the celery and mustard seeds. Add the sliced cucumbers and onions. Bring to a boil again. Boil two minutes. Using tongs, divide the pickles into 4 jars. Ladle the brine over them and seal tightly. It may look like there is not enough brine, but usually it is just the right amount. If you need more, heat equal parts honey and vinegar. These pickles may be eaten as soon as they are cooled.

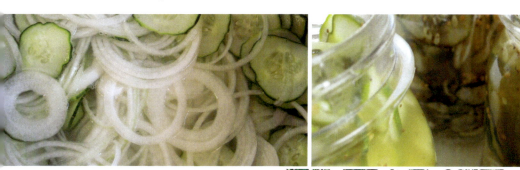

Olive Oil Pickles

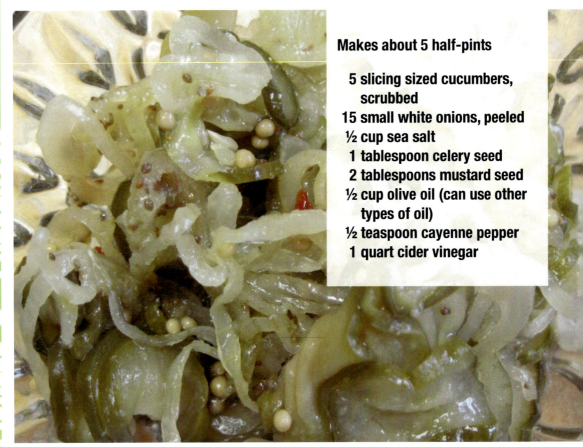

Makes about 5 half-pints

5 slicing sized cucumbers, scrubbed
15 small white onions, peeled
½ cup sea salt
1 tablespoon celery seed
2 tablespoons mustard seed
½ cup olive oil (can use other types of oil)
½ teaspoon cayenne pepper
1 quart cider vinegar

Slice the cucumber and onions very thin. The cucumbers should make 6 cups when sliced and the onions 3 cups (a 2-to-1 proportion). Mix the cucumber and onion slices together with the salt. Put them into a colander and cover with a plate topped with a heavy weight to drain overnight. Next morning, put them loosely into freshly scrubbed jars. The quantity given will make about 5 half pints. Mix together the celery and mustard seeds, oil, pepper and vinegar. Pour over the pickles in the jars. Cap and store in a cool place for several weeks. These pickles will keep as long as you can resist eating them.

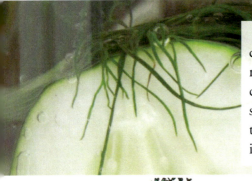

From a small cookbook by Catherine Plagemann called *Fine Preserving*, I found this unusual pickle recipe that has become a family favorite. It requires no cooking and is another one that can be made in any size batch, so it comes in handy in the fall to use up the odds and ends of cucumbers left on the vine. This is my adaptation of an old Greek recipe.

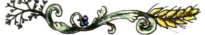

Spice of Life Specialty Foods **PRESENTS**

Dill Pickles

Makes about 7 quarts

- 6 pounds small cucumbers
- 21 cloves garlic
- 3 quarts distilled water
- 1 quart vinegar
- 1 cup pickling salt or sea salt, non-iodized
- 14 sprigs fresh dill

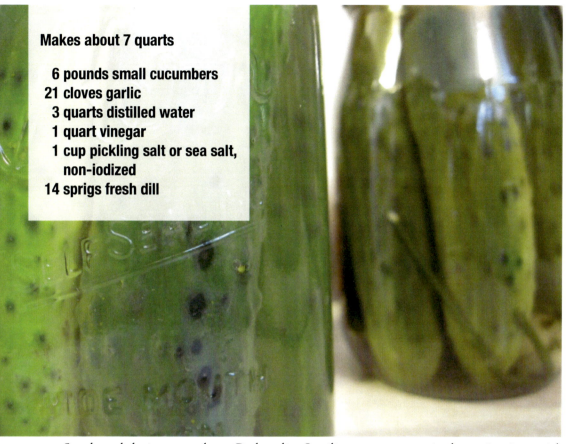

Scrub and drain cucumbers. Peel garlic. Sterilize seven quart sized canning jars, with lids and rings, upside down in boiling water. (Wide mouth jars are easiest to pack.) In another separate large kettle, boil the distilled water, vinegar, and salt for the brine. Turn the jars right side up, but leave them in the boiling water. Fill them with a sprig of dill, clove of garlic and a layer of cucumbers, tightly packed. Then put in another sprig of dill, clove of garlic and another layer of packed cucumbers. End with a third clove of garlic. Ladle boiling brine to fill the jar to the shoulder one-half inch from the top; and seal tightly. Allow the pickles to age at least one week before eating. Usually the full flavor does not develop until after a couple months.

Counter Top Dill Pickles

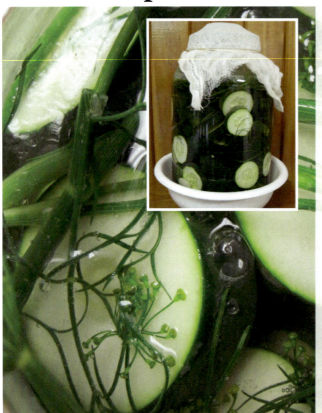

Makes a gallon of pickles

4-5 pounds small cucumbers
8-10 sprigs of dill
2 cloves garlic
8 cups water
½ cup sea salt

Naturally fermented dill pickles made without any vinegar are very easy to make. These pickles contain vitamins as well as enzymes that are helpful to digestion so they are another item in a healthy diet. They can be made with less salt or more salt as desired. These pickles can be made with odds and ends of cucumbers in large or small quantities so it is handy to make these pickles at the beginning or end of the growing season when there aren't enough cucumbers to make a full batch of other pickles.

Wash cucumbers. Cut larger cucumbers into ½-inch chunks or slices if desired. You can cut the cucumbers as you go to see how many will actually fit into your gallon container. (The chunks ripen into pickles faster than whole cucumbers.) Into a freshly scrubbed glass gallon jar or crock, put one third of the dill. Peel and slice one clove of garlic over the dill. Put half of the cucumbers in next. Repeat the layers, then top with the remaining dill. In a large kettle, boil the water and stir in the sea salt until dissolved. Allow brine to cool to room temperature; then pour over cucumber mixture. Put a small plate or plastic cover with a weight on top of the cucumbers to keep them submerged in the brine. Cover the jar with a layer of cheesecloth to keep out dust and flies. Place the jar into a shallow pan to catch any brine that overflows during fermentation. Put the whole works into a shaded corner of the counter out of the way for 3-4 days. Check the pickles daily and skim off any film or scum that forms on the surface. Taste after three days. If sufficiently pickled according to your taste, they are ready to enjoy with dinner. Remove the cheesecloth and plate, and top the jar with its cover. These pickles could also be made in a wide mouth quart-sized jar with one fourth the ingredients for a smaller quantity; although they are such good pickles, a large jarful will disappear in no time. Cover and store remainder in refrigerator for up to one month.

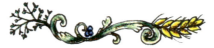

Spice of Life Specialty Foods PRESENTS

Celery Chow Chow

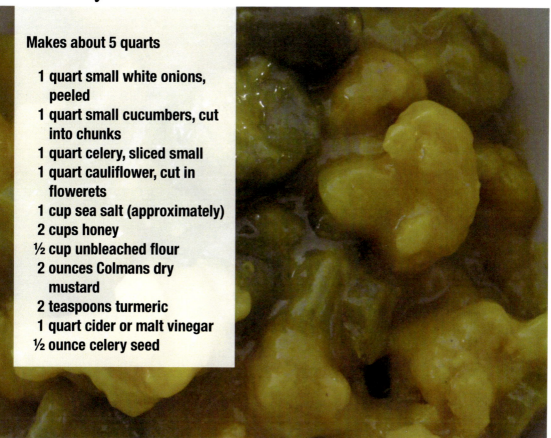

Makes about 5 quarts

- 1 quart small white onions, peeled
- 1 quart small cucumbers, cut into chunks
- 1 quart celery, sliced small
- 1 quart cauliflower, cut in flowerets
- 1 cup sea salt (approximately)
- 2 cups honey
- ½ cup unbleached flour
- 2 ounces Colmans dry mustard
- 2 teaspoons turmeric
- 1 quart cider or malt vinegar
- ½ ounce celery seed

In a large stainless, ceramic or enamel bowl, put a layer of the prepared vegetables. Sprinkle with sea salt. Add more layers of vegetables and sprinkle with salt until they are all in the bowl. Let stand overnight. In the morning, drain the brine. Rinse well and drain again. Combine the honey, flour, mustard powder, turmeric and one half of the vinegar in a large dutch oven. Boil to a cream. In another kettle, put the other half of the vinegar and the celery seed tied in a cheesecloth bag. Boil 10 minutes. Take out the bag of celery seed, and add the vinegar to the mustard sauce. Bring to a boil. Add the vegetables, and cook slowly for 20 minutes. Bottle in hot sterile jars. Seal tightly. These pickles can be eaten as soon as they cool, but, as with all pickles, their flavor improves with age.

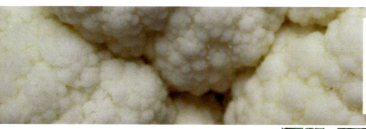

For gluten-free, substitute arrow root or tapioca starch for flour. These do thicken faster than the wheat flour.

Pickled Beets

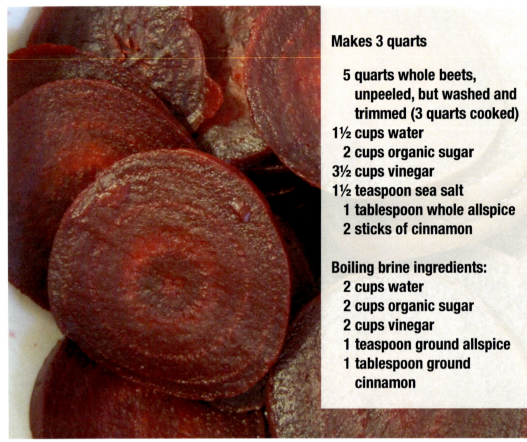

Makes 3 quarts

- 5 quarts whole beets, unpeeled, but washed and trimmed (3 quarts cooked)
- 1½ cups water
- 2 cups organic sugar
- 3½ cups vinegar
- 1½ teaspoon sea salt
- 1 tablespoon whole allspice
- 2 sticks of cinnamon

Boiling brine ingredients:
- 2 cups water
- 2 cups organic sugar
- 2 cups vinegar
- 1 teaspoon ground allspice
- 1 tablespoon ground cinnamon

Boil whole, unpeeled beets about 20 minutes until tender. Cool and rub off peels. Slice beets or cut into chunks. Put beet slices in jars. Simmer first quantities of water, sugar, vinegar, salt and spices for 15 minutes. Add second quantities of brine ingredients and bring to a boil. Pour boiling brine over beets. Break the cinnamon sticks in pieces and divide it and the whole allspice among all jars. Leave in the jars for added flavor. Seal by processing 10 minutes in a boiling water bath.

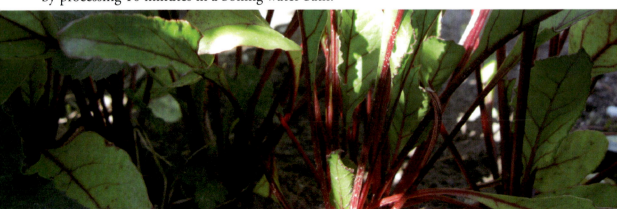

Spice of Life Specialty Foods PRESENTS

Sauerkraut

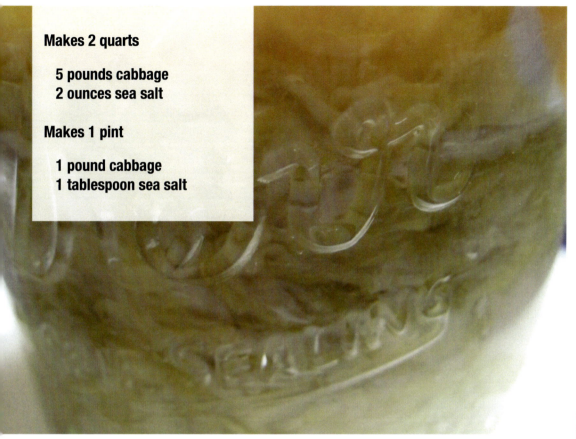

Makes 2 quarts

- 5 pounds cabbage
- 2 ounces sea salt

Makes 1 pint

- 1 pound cabbage
- 1 tablespoon sea salt

Remove outer cabbage leaves. Cut cabbage into quarters and shred finely. Using a kitchen scale, weigh the cabbage in a stainless steel bowl. Then add the sea salt and mix well. Pack the cabbage/salt mixture tightly into two clean, wide mouth quart sized jars or a two-quart crock. Push down hard when packing the jars so that the cabbage juice rises above the cabbage. The juice will run over the top of the jar, so work over a pan that will catch the drips. Save some of that juice in another jar to use later. When the jars are full, cut a small plastic disc (from a plastic container lid) to fit inside the top of the jar and hold the cabbage submerged in the brine. Cover the jars with cheesecloth held on with a rubber band. Set the sauerkraut in a cool, shaded corner of the counter. Check it daily, and skim off any scum that forms. Rinse the cheesecloth daily. If brine level falls below the top of the cabbage during fermentation, add some juice from the jar that you saved earlier. The sauerkraut should be done in 10 to 12 days. Then it can be packed into smaller canning jars and processed in a boiling water bath, or it can be kept refrigerated.

Basic Tomato Sauce

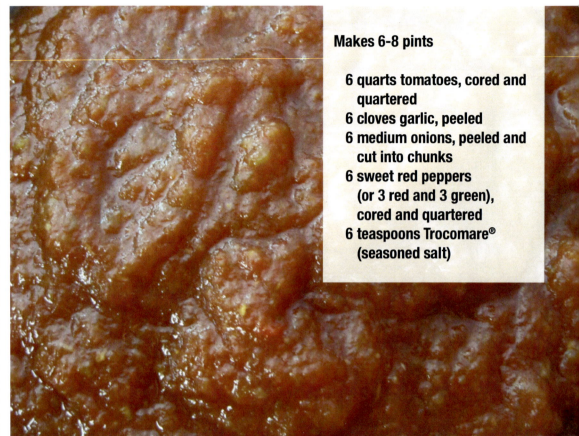

Makes 6-8 pints

- 6 quarts tomatoes, cored and quartered
- 6 cloves garlic, peeled
- 6 medium onions, peeled and cut into chunks
- 6 sweet red peppers (or 3 red and 3 green), cored and quartered
- 6 teaspoons Trocomare® (seasoned salt)

In a large dutch oven or stock pot, put all ingredients, except the Trocomare®. Heat over medium heat, stirring occasionally and cook until vegetables are tender enough to go through a food mill or ricer to remove tomato skins and seeds. Return to heat and cook gently until the volume is down by about half of the original. Season with Trocomare® to taste. Fill pint jars, cap and process in boiling water bath for 25 minutes to seal. Cool and store for use in your favorite recipes.

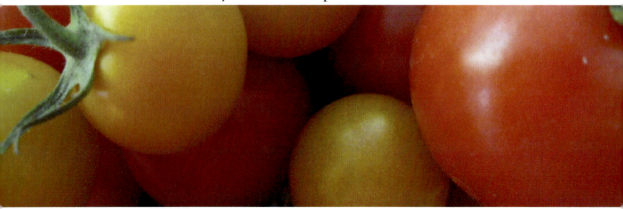

Spice of Life Specialty Foods PRESENTS

Victoria's Salsa

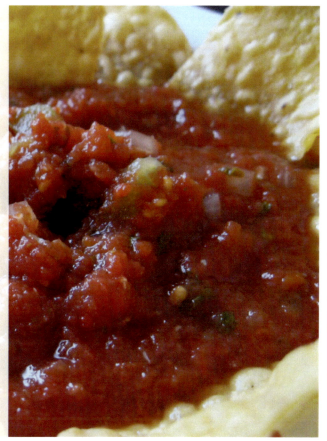

Makes about 10 pints

Initial sauce:
- 30 tomatoes
- 2 large onions, quartered
- 1 green pepper, seeded and quartered
- 1 sweet red pepper, seeded and quartered
- 4 cloves garlic
- 2 jalapeños

Chunky ingredients:
- 10 tomatoes
- 1 onion, chopped
- 2 cloves garlic, minced
- 1 red pepper, diced
- 1 green pepper, diced
- 2-3 jalapeños
- 12 ounces tomato paste
- 1 cup cider vinegar
- ⅓ cup Trocomare® (seasoned salt)
- 1 teaspoon oregano
- ¼ cup lemon juice
- 1 bunch cilantro, chopped

Put tomatoes, onions, peppers, garlic, and jalapeños in a pot for the initial sauce. Cook until reduced by half. Run through a food mill to remove skins and seeds. Return to kettle and heat. In a separate pot, scald tomatoes in boiling water to remove skins. Cool and cube tomatoes and add to sauce along with the rest of the ingredients. Heat to boiling. Pack into hot, clean canning jars and seal.

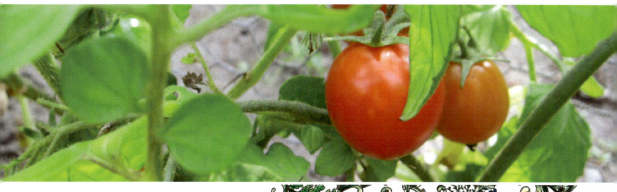

Whole Cranberry Sauce

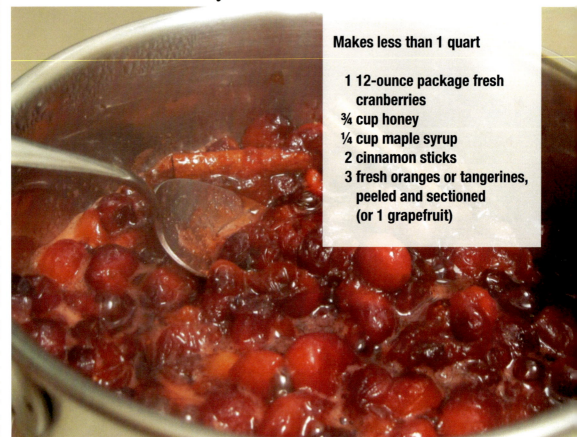

Makes less than 1 quart

- 1 12-ounce package fresh cranberries
- ¾ cup honey
- ¼ cup maple syrup
- 2 cinnamon sticks
- 3 fresh oranges or tangerines, peeled and sectioned (or 1 grapefruit)

Sort cranberries and cook with honey and maple syrup in a medium saucepan over medium high heat, stirring occasionally to prevent scorching or boil over, until most of the berries have popped, about 10 minutes. Add cinnamon sticks and orange sections. Cover and cool. This sauce may be served warm or cold but is best if made a few days ahead to let the cinnamon flavor permeate the mixture.

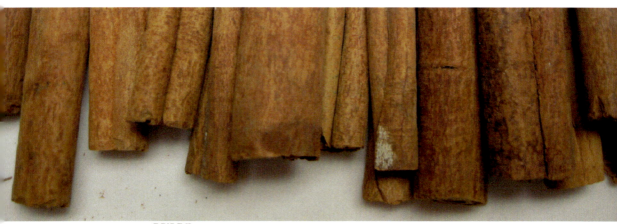

Spice of Life Specialty Foods PRESENTS

Berry Sauce: for waffles, etc.

Makes more than 1 quart

- 4 cups frozen (or fresh) wild blueberries
- ½ cup maple syrup
- ¼ cup honey
- 3 tablespoons arrowroot starch
- water to dissolve starch
- 1 tablespoon butter
- 1 teaspoon vanilla
- 1 cup frozen (or fresh) raspberries

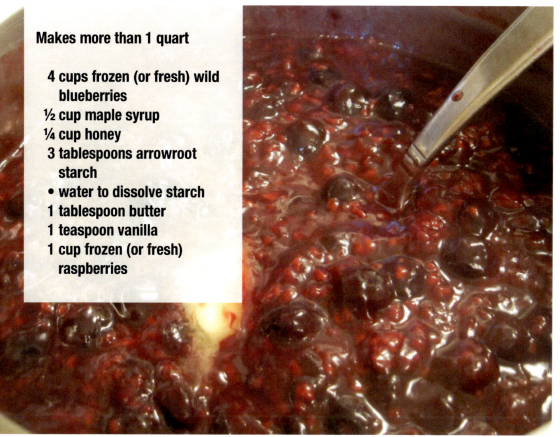

Put blueberries into a saucepan with maple syrup and honey. Bring to a boil. Cook for 5 minutes. Remove blueberries from heat. In a cup, add enough water to the arrowroot starch to dissolve; mix to a smooth cream. Add mixed starch to blueberries and stir constantly until thickened. Add butter, and mix in until melted. Then add vanilla, and stir again. Finally, mix in frozen raspberries. The heat of the sauce will thaw them. Serve with pancakes, waffles, or as a dessert sauce.

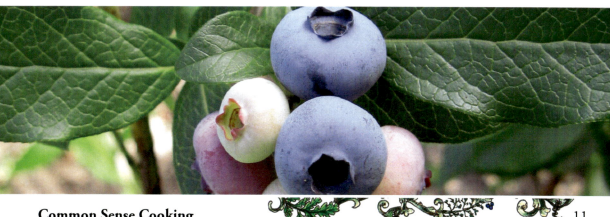

Low/Alternate Sugar Jam or Jelly

Now you can make sugar-free jams and jellies using the "low-methoxyl" or LM pectin that doesn't require sugar to jell. This pectin sets up in the presence of calcium. Some fruits contain enough of their own calcium for jelling but others don't so, to be sure, a packet of (tasteless) di-calcium phosphate is included when you purchase this pectin. LM pectin allows a person to make jam using honey, maple syrup, or concentrated fruit juice for sweetening or no sweetener at all. Also the fruits need not be boiled to death in this jam because LM pectin requires only a low boiling point to jell. If you choose to make jam with a low sugar content using LM pectin, you must either hot pack seal or freeze the jam to preserve it. Bottle it in small enough jars so that once the jam is opened it will be used within two weeks. Low-methoxyl pectin can be purchased as Pomona's Universal Pectin from the grocery store or by mail order from Walnut Acres, Penns Creek, PA 17862.

To make the jam or jelly:

Prepare the fruit; clean the berries and mash if desired. Also, strain to remove seeds if desired. For jelly, boil the fruit and drip the juice from the pulp through a cloth bag. Measure the fruit or juice into a heavy bottomed kettle.

Prepare calcium solution by putting ½ teaspoon di-calcium phosphate into ½ cup water in a jar with a tight fitting lid. Shake well.

The LM pectin can be either mixed with honey or maple syrup using ⅛ cup sweetener and ½ teaspoon dry pectin for each cup of fruit or juice. Or 2 tablespoons of the LM pectin can be dissolved in 1 pint of very hot water in the blender by blending on high speed for several minutes. Use ¼ cup of this solution per cup of fruit or juice. The extra solution can be stored in the refrigerator for future use. Measure and use in jellied form.

Sterilize the jars and lids ready for the jam.

Bring fruit or juice to a boil. Add the pectin mixture. If using the liquid pectin solution, remember to add desired sweetener using ¼ cup per cup of fruit or berries (more or less as desired). Bring again to a full rolling boil while stirring to dissolve all the pectin.

Now add to the boiling fruit ¾ teaspoon of the di-calcium solution after shaking well. Stir well to mix and pour into sterilized jars and seal. If desired, before bottling, test a small amount of jam on a saucer in the freezer to see that the consistency is as desired when cooled. If the jam is too runny, add another ½ teaspoon of the calcium solution.

Small batches of jam can also be made using arrowroot powder or kuzu starch to thicken. This jam also would need to be refrigerated or frozen to preserve it.

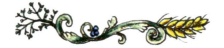

Spice of Life Specialty Foods PRESENTS

Wild Blackberry Jelly

Makes 2 ½ pints

- 4 cups blackberry juice
- 1 cup honey
- 2 teaspoons low methoxyl pectin (Pomona's Universal Pectin is one brand)
- 1 tablespoon di-calcium phosphate solution

Put 3 pints or 5 half-pint jars with caps to sterilize in boiling water. In a large kettle, heat the juice with ½ cup of honey. Mix the pectin with the rest of the honey, then add it to the juice. Bring the juice to a boil and stir until the pectin dissolves. Then add the calcium solution, and mix well. If desired, put a small amount of jelly on a saucer chilled from the freezer to check the consistency. If it is too thin at room temperature, add more calcium solution. The jelly should be ready to put into sterile jars and seal. When sealed, the jelly will keep a year. After opening, the jelly will need to be used within a couple of weeks. Always store opened jelly in the refrigerator because of its lower sugar content.

Many uninhabited areas in the Keweenaw area of Michigan are rich with wild blackberries, chokecherries, and even currants. These fruits make wonderful jelly that is low in cost. As you pick these berries, save them in the freezer until you have a large amount. Then cook them in a large kettle over medium-low heat to extract the juice. Drain the juice from the pulp using an old pillowcase or other large clean cloth. Hang it above a bowl to drip over night. Then measure the juice to be used in these recipes.

Currant Jelly

Makes 3 pints

- 4 cups currant juice
- 2 cups honey
- 1 tablespoon pectin
- 1 tablespoon di-calcium phosphate solution

Follow same directions as for making the blackberry jelly.

The recipes may be doubled. The general rule is to use ⅛ cup honey and ½ teaspoon dry pectin for each cup of fruit juice. Tart berries require a larger amount of honey than sweet ones. Di-calcium phosphate and directions come with the pectin when you purchase it.

PICKLES & PRESERVES

Common Sense Cooking

Pepperidge Farm Style Apricot Jam

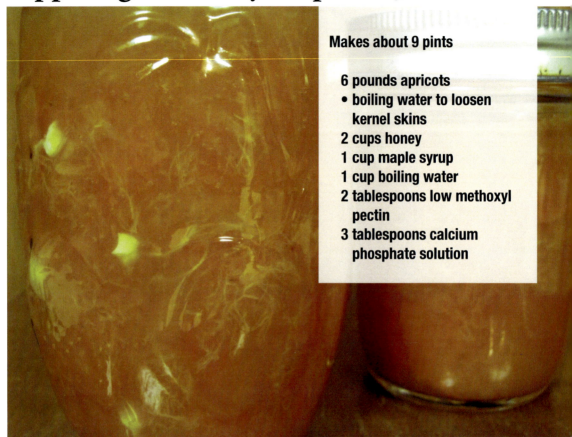

Makes about 9 pints

- 6 pounds apricots
- boiling water to loosen kernel skins
- 2 cups honey
- 1 cup maple syrup
- 1 cup boiling water
- 2 tablespoons low methoxyl pectin
- 3 tablespoons calcium phosphate solution

Split the apricots and save the pits. Take the pits to a cement floor. Hit them with a hammer, one at a time, as you would crack a nut. Save the kernels. Pour boiling water over them to loosen the skins. After about 5 minutes, pinch off the brown skins and save the nut meats. Put the apricot fruit in a large kettle with the honey and syrup. Bring to a boil, and cook about 5 minutes, squashing the apricots using a potato masher. Put 1 cup boiling water in blender, add pectin and blend at low speed until dissolved. Add pectin mixture to jam; stir in. Add calcium phosphate solution and kernels; mix well. If desired, put a spoonful of jam on a saucer in the freezer to check the consistency when cool. Bottle the jam while hot in sterile jars capped with sterile lids and rings.

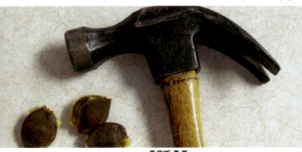
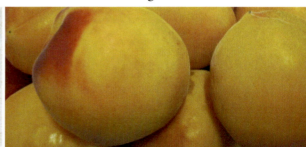

Spice of Life Specialty Foods PRESENTS

Fluffy Millet Side Dish

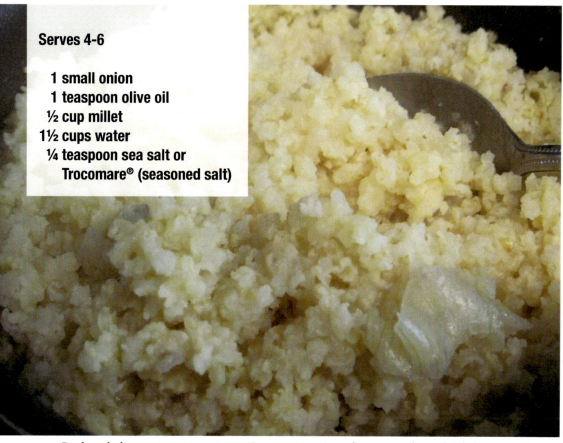

Serves 4-6

- 1 small onion
- 1 teaspoon olive oil
- ½ cup millet
- 1½ cups water
- ¼ teaspoon sea salt or Trocomare® (seasoned salt)

Peel and slice onion into rings. Saute onion in oil over medium high heat until slightly browned. Add millet and sauté while stirring to toast lightly. Add water and salt. Bring to a boil. Then lower heat, cover and allow to cook gently for half an hour. Serve as a side dish with fish or beans.

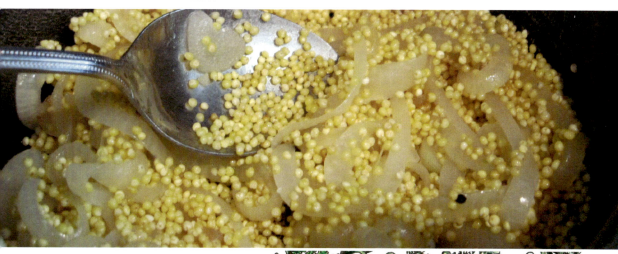

Common Sense Cooking

Buckwheat Kasha

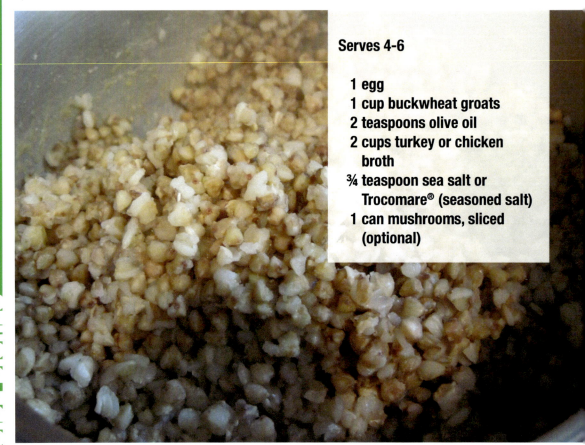

Serves 4-6

1 egg
1 cup buckwheat groats
2 teaspoons olive oil
2 cups turkey or chicken broth
¾ teaspoon sea salt or Trocomare® (seasoned salt)
1 can mushrooms, sliced (optional)

In a small mixing bowl, mix the raw egg with the buckwheat groats until all kernels are coated. In a two quart saucepan that has a lid, heat the oil over medium high heat. Put in the buckwheat and egg mixture and stir to cook the egg coating around each kernel. Add broth and salt. Bring to a boil. Add mushrooms if using. Lower heat, cover and cook gently for half an hour. If made with homemade broth containing chunks of meat, this can be served as a main dish. Without meat, serve as a side dish.

Variation: Use 2 cups water in place of broth and substitute vegetable bouillon for the salt.

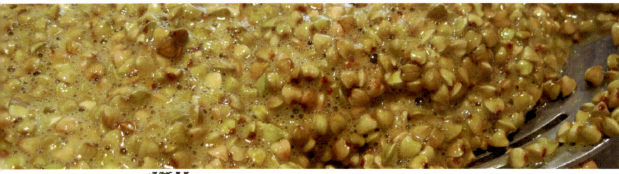

Spice of Life Specialty Foods PRESENTS

Bread Stuffing

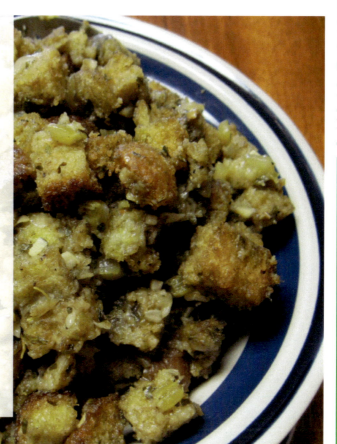

Serves 8-10

- 2 cups onions, chopped
- 3 cups celery, chopped
- 2 cloves garlic, minced
- 2 tablespoons butter or oil
- 1 cup water
- 12 cups dry bread cubes
- 1 tablespoon parsley
- 1/8 teaspoon red pepper, crushed
- 1/4 teaspoon oregano
- 1 teaspoon ground savory
- 1 teaspoon sage
- 2 teaspoons marjoram
- 2 teaspoons thyme
- 1 teaspoon ground rosemary
- 1 teaspoon sea salt or Trocomare® (seasoned salt)

Saute the onions, celery, and garlic in the butter or oil. Then add water; cover and cook 10 minutes. In a large mixing bowl, mix together the bread cubes with the seasonings and salt. When the celery is almost tender, add the vegetables to the bread cubes, and mix well. If using dry cubes from home made or whole grain bread, add 1-2 cups more water to soften the bread cubes. The stuffing should be moist but not soggy. Stuff the crop of the turkey first, and fasten the neck skin with a metal skewer. Then fill the main cavity of the turkey. I like to put a piece of baking parchment or cheesecloth in the back of the turkey so the stuffing can be easily removed after baking.

Note: You can use a good poultry seasoning instead of the above herb combination.

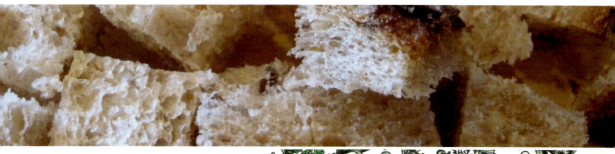

Rice Stuffing

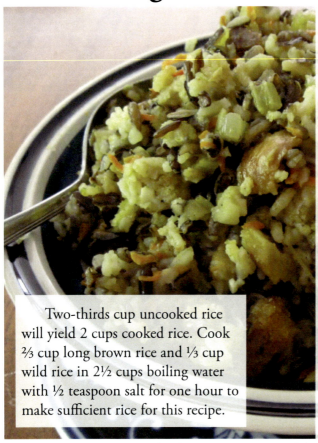

Serves 8-10

2½ cups water
½ teaspoon sea salt
⅓ cup wild rice
⅔ cup long grain brown rice
1 cup onion, chopped
1 cup celery, chopped
½ cup carrot, grated
1 clove garlic, minced
4 tablespoons butter
   (½ stick/¼ cup)
1 tablespoon vegetable broth
   powder
½ cup hot water
1 teaspoon poultry seasoning
4 cups whole wheat bread
   cubes, toasted or dry
2 teaspoons sea salt or
   Trocomare® (seasoned salt)

Two-thirds cup uncooked rice will yield 2 cups cooked rice. Cook ⅔ cup long brown rice and ⅓ cup wild rice in 2½ cups boiling water with ½ teaspoon salt for one hour to make sufficient rice for this recipe.

In a medium saucepan, boil 2 ½ cups water. Add salt and rice. Reduce heat to medium-low, cover and simmer for 50 minutes. In a large skillet, saute the onion, celery carrots, and garlic in butter until tender. Dissolve the broth powder in ½ cup hot water. Add to vegetables in skillet along with rice and seasoning. Stir to mix. Add the bread cubes and two additional teaspoons of salt. Mix again until well blended. Use to stuff a small turkey or turkey roast. Double the recipe for a 12-pound turkey.

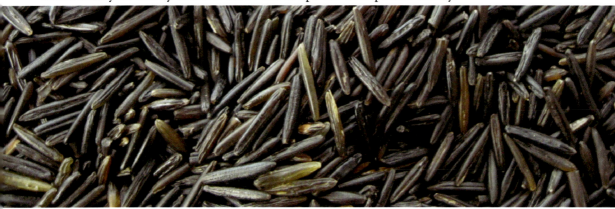

Spice of Life Specialty Foods PRESENTS

Allspiced Cider

Makes 6-8 cups

- 1 tablespoon whole allspice
- 3 cups apple cider
- 1 3-inch cinnamon stick
- 1 cup orange juice, freshly squeezed
- 1 lemon, sliced
- 2 teaspoons honey

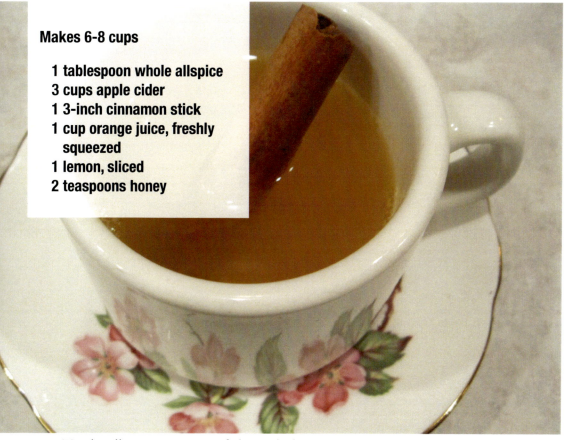

Tie the allspice in a piece of cheesecloth or tea strainer. Combine the cider, cinnamon, allspice, orange juice, lemon slices, and honey in a medium saucepan. Bring to a boil. Simmer covered for 5 minutes. Remove spice bag and serve.

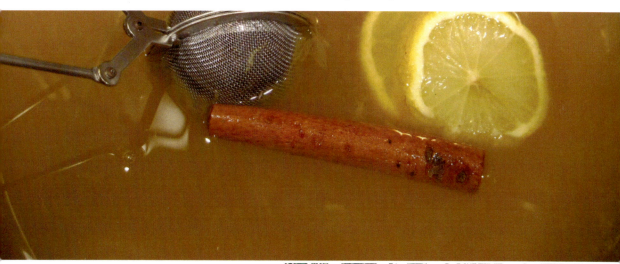

Nori Rolls (Sushi)

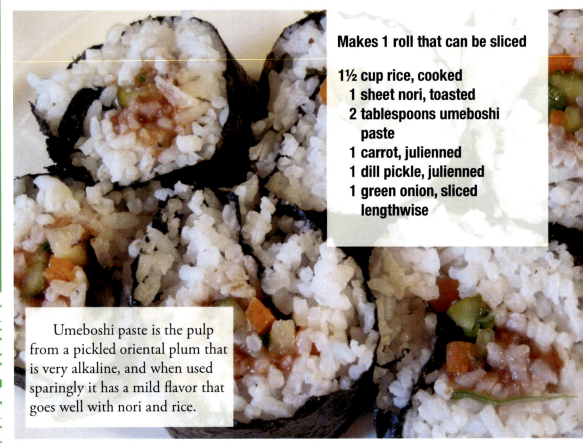

Makes 1 roll that can be sliced

1½ cup rice, cooked
1 sheet nori, toasted
2 tablespoons umeboshi paste
1 carrot, julienned
1 dill pickle, julienned
1 green onion, sliced lengthwise

Umeboshi paste is the pulp from a pickled oriental plum that is very alkaline, and when used sparingly it has a mild flavor that goes well with nori and rice.

SIDE DISHES

Spread cooked rice over a sheet of nori leaving about a half inch uncovered at the top and bottom. Spread a line of umeboshi paste across rice about ¼ inch wide. Place a few pieces of carrots, pickles, and green onion on top of the umeboshi line. Roll the nori as you would a jelly roll or cinnamon roll dough. Cut into 2-inch thick slices and serve.

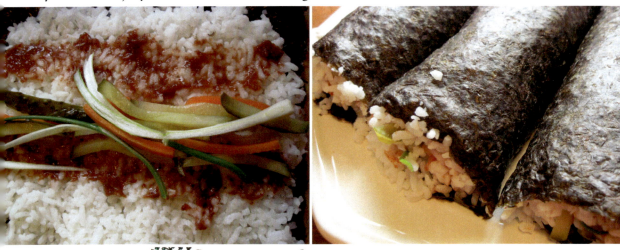

Spice of Life Specialty Foods PRESENTS

Savory Scalloped Potatoes

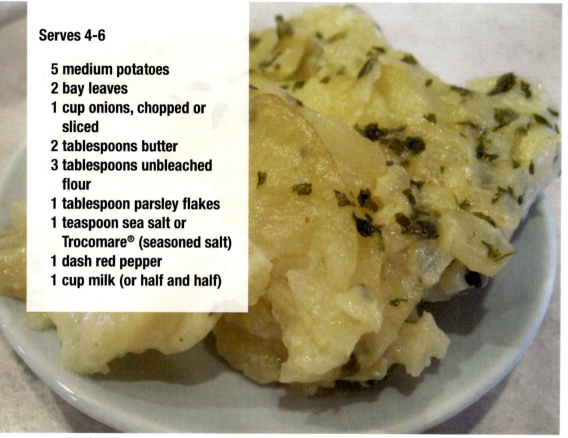

Serves 4-6

- 5 medium potatoes
- 2 bay leaves
- 1 cup onions, chopped or sliced
- 2 tablespoons butter
- 3 tablespoons unbleached flour
- 1 tablespoon parsley flakes
- 1 teaspoon sea salt or Trocomare® (seasoned salt)
- 1 dash red pepper
- 1 cup milk (or half and half)

Scrub or peel and slice enough potatoes to make 5 cups. Put one bay leaf in bottom of 2 quart covered casserole dish. Put potato slices in. In a sauce pan, saute onions in butter until translucent. It doesn't matter if the onions brown slightly. Stir in the flour, parsley, salt and a dash of red pepper. Mix in milk. Cook, while stirring until milk starts to thicken. Remove from heat and pour over potatoes. Put remaining bay leaf on top; cover casserole. Bake at 400° for 1 hour and 15 minutes or until potatoes are done. Casserole may be stirred during baking to mix onions in. Remove top bay leaf before serving. Serve as a side dish as is, or top with cheese in the last 5 minutes of baking to use as a main dish.

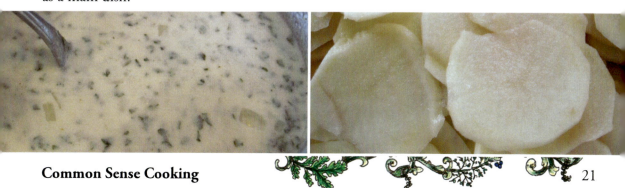

Common Sense Cooking

Chicken Vegetable Soup

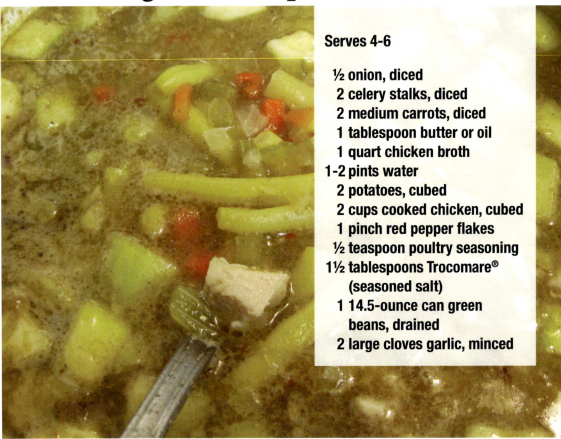

Serves 4-6

- ½ onion, diced
- 2 celery stalks, diced
- 2 medium carrots, diced
- 1 tablespoon butter or oil
- 1 quart chicken broth
- 1-2 pints water
- 2 potatoes, cubed
- 2 cups cooked chicken, cubed
- 1 pinch red pepper flakes
- ½ teaspoon poultry seasoning
- 1½ tablespoons Trocomare® (seasoned salt)
- 1 14.5-ounce can green beans, drained
- 2 large cloves garlic, minced

Use a three quart pot. Sauté the chopped onion, celery, and carrots in butter until onions are translucent. (The juice in the canned beans can be used as water for the soup.) Add chicken broth, water, and potatoes. Boil for 10 minutes. While boiling, cut the chicken and mix with the red pepper flakes, poultry seasoning and Trocomare®. Drop the temperature on the soup and add the chicken, drained beans, and garlic. Simmer for 10 minutes. Soup can be reheated in crock pot, and broth added as necessary.

Fresh beans can be used in place of canned. Simmer until the beans are cooked.

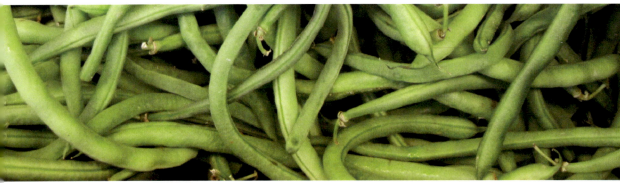

Spice of Life Specialty Foods PRESENTS

Chicken Noodle Soup

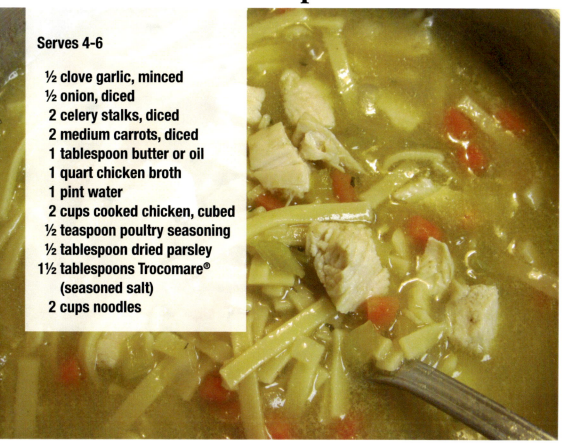

Serves 4-6

½ clove garlic, minced
½ onion, diced
2 celery stalks, diced
2 medium carrots, diced
1 tablespoon butter or oil
1 quart chicken broth
1 pint water
2 cups cooked chicken, cubed
½ teaspoon poultry seasoning
½ tablespoon dried parsley
1½ tablespoons Trocomare®
   (seasoned salt)
2 cups noodles

Use a three quart pot. Sauté garlic, onion, celery and carrots in butter until onions are translucent. Add broth, water, chicken, poultry seasoning, parsley, and Trocomare®. Bring to a boil and add noodles. Boil for 10 minutes. Continue to simmer until noodles are done. Soup can be reheated in crock pot, and broth added as necessary.

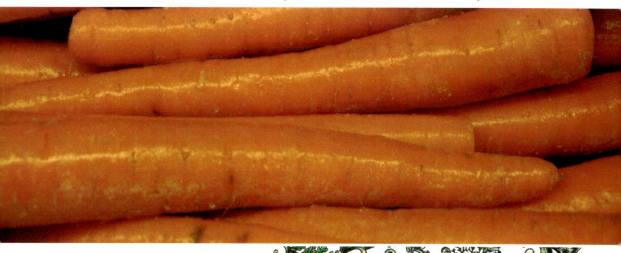

Heart Warming Turkey Soup

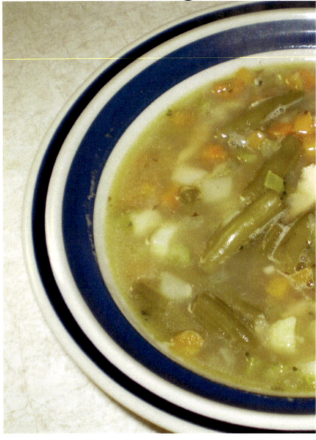

Serves 4-6

- 1 medium onion
- 2 stalks celery
- 1 small garlic clove
- 1 tablespoon olive oil or turkey fat
- 1 quart turkey broth
- 1 cup cooked turkey chunks
- 1 piece kombu sea vegetable (about 4 inches)
- 1 carrot
- 2 potatoes
- 1 cup of fresh vegetables: green beans, broccoli, cauliflower, peas, or corn
- 1 tablespoon parsley flakes
- 1-2 teaspoons Trocomare® (seasoned salt), according to taste
- 1 shake red pepper flakes
- ½ teaspoon poultry seasoning

Peel and chop the onion. Chop celery and garlic. Saute the onion, celery, and garlic in oil (or turkey fat if the turkey is organically grown). Add the broth with meat pieces and kombu and bring to a boil. Scrub and cut the carrot into attractive pieces. Scrub and peel the potatoes as desired. Cut the potato into bite-sized pieces. Add to soup. Then add any other vegetables that are on hand. Cook at medium heat for about 15 minutes until vegetables are tender. Remove the kombu; cut it into ½ inch squares and put back into soup. Last add parsley and seasonings. Serve hot with whole grain bread.

If the turkey broth has no flavor of poultry seasoning from stuffing, add a pinch each of thyme, savory, rosemary, sage, oregano, and marjoram to the soup at the end of the cooking time.

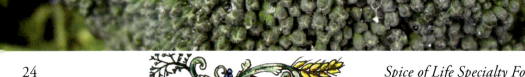

Spice of Life Specialty Foods PRESENTS

Split Pea Soup

Serves 4-6

- 1 cup green split peas
- 4 cups water
- 1 4-inch piece wakame sea vegetable
- 1 onion, sliced
- 4 large carrots, peeled and cut into cubes
- 1 teaspoon thyme
- 1 teaspoon sea salt, OR 4 tablespoons miso

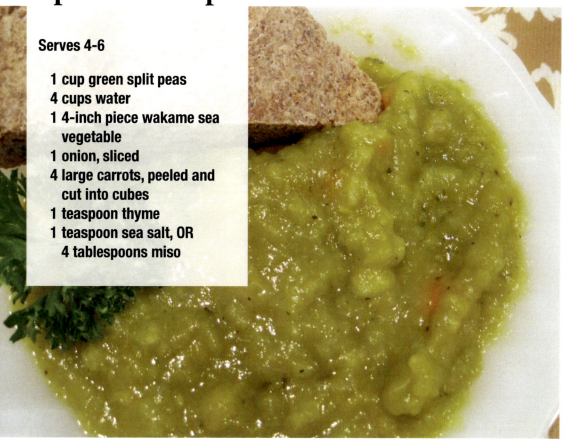

Put peas into large kettle with water and wakame. Bring to a boil. Add onion and carrots. Reduce heat, cover and cook for 3 hours, stirring occasionally. Before serving, season with thyme and salt or miso. If using miso, ladle out one cup of the soup broth into small bowl. Dissolve the miso paste in the broth and pour it back into the soup. Stir to mix well and serve immediately. Pea soup goes very well with rye bread or Scandinavian style rye hardtack.

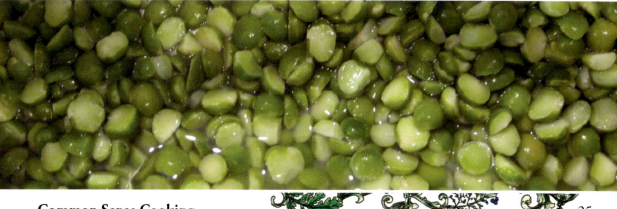

Common Sense Cooking

Basic Miso Soup

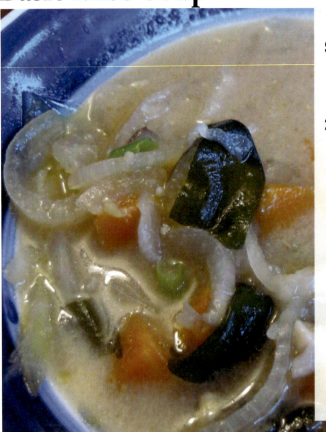

Serves 4

1 medium onion, peeled and sliced in rings
2-3 drops sesame oil
3 cups water
1 carrot, scrubbed or peeled and cut into triangular pieces
½ cup cabbage, sliced thin
1 shiitake mushroom cap, soaked and chopped (optional—or use fresh mushroom)
1 piece of wakame sea vegetable (3 inches long)
2 tablespoons barley miso paste
1 green onion, sliced

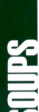

In a 2 quart saucepan, saute the onion in a few drops of sesame oil for 3 minutes. Add the water and vegetables. Crumble the wakame into small pieces before adding. Bring to a boil. Reduce heat, cover and cook about 10 minutes until the vegetables are tender. Remove 1/2 cup of the broth into a small bowl. Dissolve the miso paste in the broth; then add this back to the soup. Garnish with sliced green onions. Serve hot.

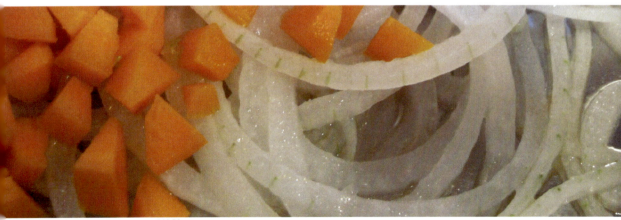

Spice of Life Specialty Foods PRESENTS

Hunter's Stew

Serves 8

- 1 pound lean venison, cut in ½ inch cubes
- 1 small onion, cut fine
- ½ cup celery, chopped
- 1 tablespoon butter or oil
- 2 or more cups water, depending on vegetables below
- 3 bouillon cubes, beef or vegetable
- 1 bay leaf
- ¼ teaspoon sweet basil
- 4 medium potatoes, peeled and cubed, OR
- ¼ pound fine noodles
- 1 pint canned tomatoes
- 1 pint canned peas (OR 1½ cups frozen)
- 1 pint canned corn (OR 1½ cups frozen)
- Trocomare® (seasoned salt) and pepper to taste

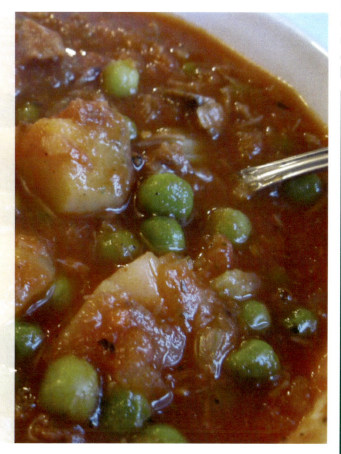

In a large kettle, saute the meat, onion and celery in butter or oil until meat and onions are browned. Add water, bouillon, spices and potatoes or pasta. Bring to a boil. Reduce heat, but keep simmering for one-half hour. Then add tomatoes (tomato sauce will give the stew a red color), peas, and corn. Check for seasonings, and add Trocomare® and pepper if desired. Serve with whole grain bread or crackers.

Note: Your natural food store should have vegetable bouillon cubes that are made without MSG. If using canned vegetables, include the liquid from the cans. If using frozen vegetables, add an additional cup of water to broth.

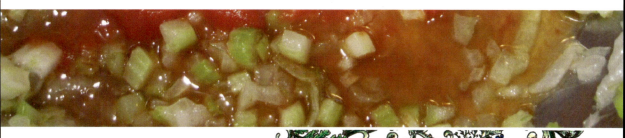

Common Sense Cooking

Beef Chili

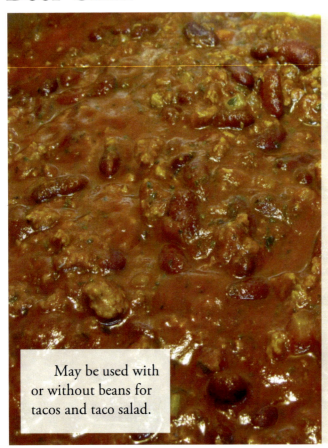

Serves 4-6

- 1 pound lean ground beef
- ½ cup onion, chopped
- 1 rib of celery, finely chopped
- 2 15-ounce cans tomato sauce
- 1 2-inch strip of red and green sweet pepper if the tomato sauce does not contain it
- 2 15-ounce cans dark red kidney beans
- ¼ cup maple syrup
- 1 tablespoon Trocomare® (seasoned salt)
- 1 tablespoon dried parsley
- 1 tablespoon dried basil
- 2-3 teaspoons chili powder, depending on how hot you like it
- 1 large clove garlic, minced

May be used with or without beans for tacos and taco salad.

Brown the ground beef over medium-high heat. Add chopped onion and celery to the beef. Saute until translucent. Add tomato sauce. If the tomato sauce does not contain green and red sweet peppers, then blend a small portion of sauce with a two-inch strip of both red and green pepper before putting into the chili. Rinse and drain kidney beans, and add them to chili. Then add maple syrup, Trocomare®, parsley, basil, and chili powder. Allow to simmer for 15-20 minutes. Put in garlic and taste for seasonings.

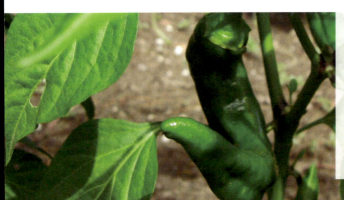

When you roast a larger amount of meat—beef, lamb or turkey, you can freeze some of the leftovers along with some of the pan juice in the same container. Then when you come to use them, reheat in the juice in a low over about 200°. The meat tastes as though freshly roasted.

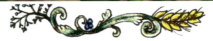

Spice of Life Specialty Foods PRESENTS

Baked Beans

Serves 8-10

- 2 cups white navy beans
- 1 piece kombu sea vegetable
- 1 teaspoon sea salt
- ⅓ cup maple syrup
- ¼ cup organic ketchup
- ½ teaspoon ginger
- 1½ teaspoon mustard powder
- 1 dash crushed red pepper (optional)

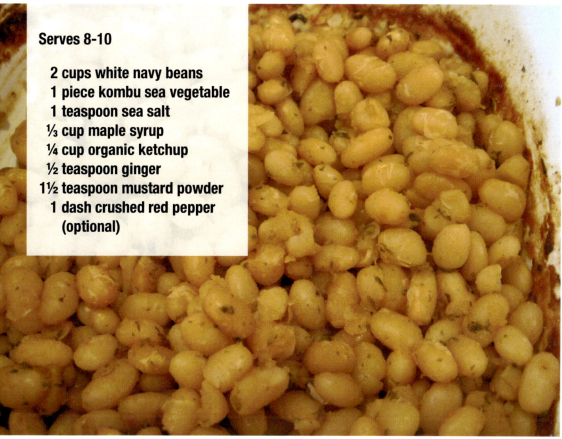

Wash and drain the beans. Put into large kettle, add kombu and cover with water. Bring to a boil. Reduce heat, cover and simmer 45 minutes. Reserve 1 ½ cups bean liquid and mix with salt, syrup, ketchup, ginger, mustard, and red pepper. Put beans and kombu into 2 quart covered casserole dish. Pour seasoning liquid over beans. Cover and bake for 3 hours at 325°. Stir occasionally and add more water if needed.

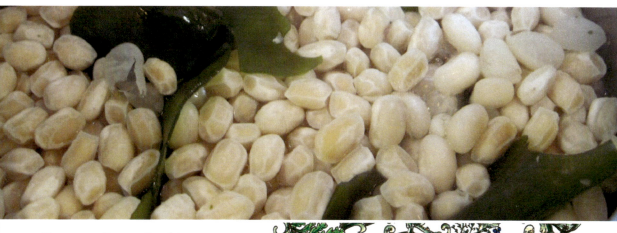

Common Sense Cooking

Basic Blender Mayonnaise

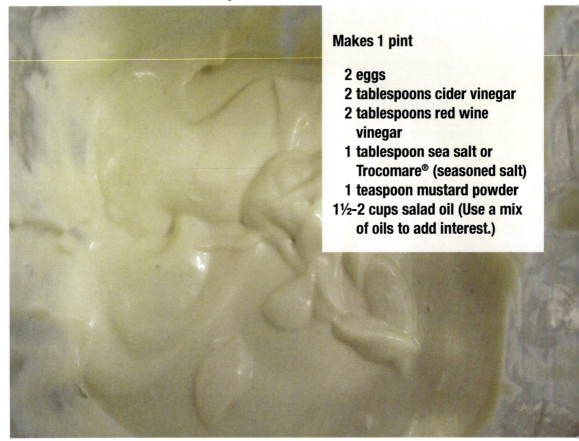

Makes 1 pint

- 2 eggs
- 2 tablespoons cider vinegar
- 2 tablespoons red wine vinegar
- 1 tablespoon sea salt or Trocomare® (seasoned salt)
- 1 teaspoon mustard powder
- 1½-2 cups salad oil (Use a mix of oils to add interest.)

Put eggs, vinegar, salt, and mustard powder into blender. Cover and process at medium speed. Then increase the speed to high; pour in the oil in a slow, steady stream. When the mayonnaise thickens, the oil will want to stay on top, so you will have to stop the blender, and use a rubber spatula to push the oil down to the bottom. Continue to process while stopping occasionally to mix the oil as needed until thick. Mayonnaise will thicken more in the refrigerator.

Homemade mayonnaise is handy to have on hand. It can be used as the base for other salad dressing, dips and sauces. When you add to it chopped sweet pickles and green onions, you have tartar sauce to serve with fish. Sweetened with honey or maple syrup, mayonnaise makes a good dressing for coleslaw or waldorf salad.

Mayonnaise can be made from scratch quickly and easily, especially with the blender. I have had better success making blender mayonnaise with cold ingredients rather than letting them warm to room temperature as the instruction books say.

Spice of Life Specialty Foods PRESENTS

Italian Style Salad Dressing

Makes about ¾ cup

- ⅓ cup vinegar or fresh lemon juice
- ½ cup olive or other salad oil
- 2 teaspoons sea salt or Trocomare® (seasoned salt)
- 1 tablespoon honey or maple syrup (optional)
- 1 large clove garlic, minced
- 1 green onion, chopped fine
- ¾ inch strip of sweet red pepper, minced
- 1 pinch of parsley, finely crushed
- 1 pinch of oregano, finely crushed
- 1 pinch of basil, finely crushed

Combine all ingredients in a covered jar and shake well. Allow flavors to blend for several hours before using.

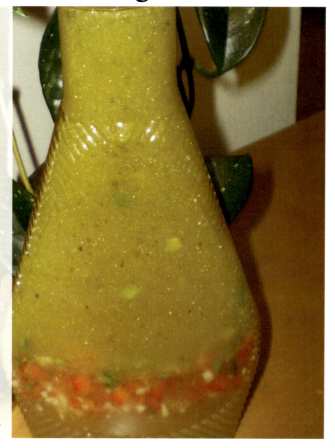

Homemade Blue Cheese Salad Dressing

Makes about 1 cup

- ½ cup plain Greek yogurt or sour cream
- ¼ cup homemade mayonnaise (see recipe on page 30)
- 1 tablespoon fresh squeezed lemon juice
- ⅓ cup crumbled blue cheese
- 1 small clove fresh garlic, peeled
- 1 tablespoon fine grated Parmesan cheese

Put all ingredients into blender or food processor and blend until smooth. You may need to stop occasionally to push the dressing down from sides of blender. Chill before serving.

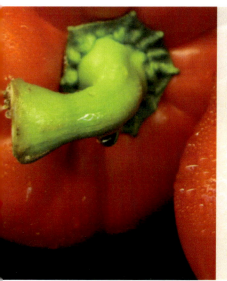

Elsie's Cream Cheese Salad Dressing

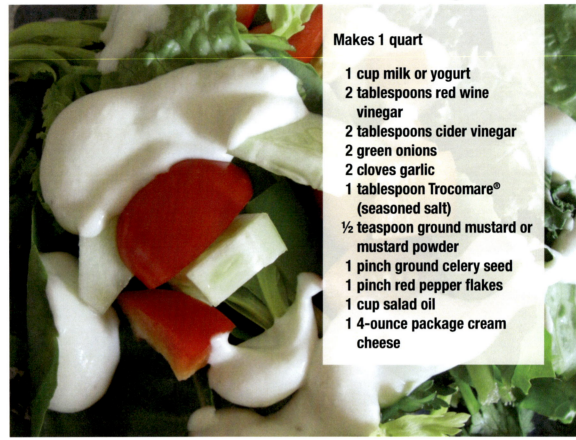

Makes 1 quart

- 1 cup milk or yogurt
- 2 tablespoons red wine vinegar
- 2 tablespoons cider vinegar
- 2 green onions
- 2 cloves garlic
- 1 tablespoon Trocomare® (seasoned salt)
- ½ teaspoon ground mustard or mustard powder
- 1 pinch ground celery seed
- 1 pinch red pepper flakes
- 1 cup salad oil
- 1 4-ounce package cream cheese

Put milk in blender. Add vinegar, onion, garlic, seasonings. Blend. Pour in oil while blending. Then add cream cheese a piece at a time, and blend until smooth. Refrigerate to allow flavors to blend. For dip, double amount of cream cheese.

Original recipe is from Elsie Muonio.

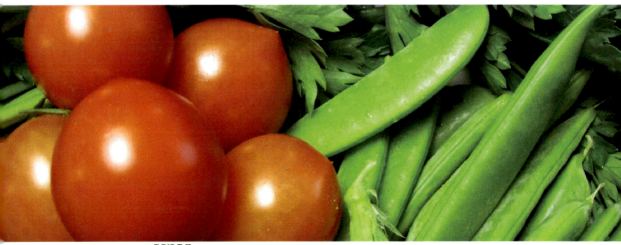

Spice of Life Specialty Foods PRESENTS

French Garden Salad (Salade Niçoise)

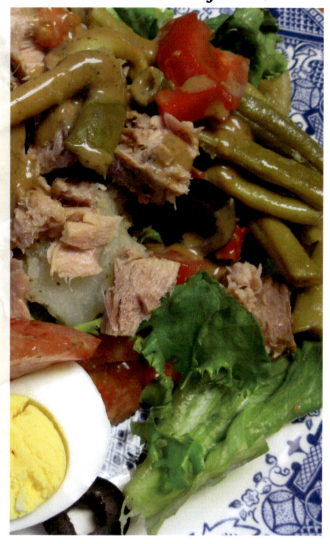

Serves 4

- 2 large potatoes
- 1 pound green beans
- 4 eggs
- 1 slice sweet onion
- 1 head romaine or other leaf lettuce
- 2 ripe tomatoes
- ½ sweet red pepper
- ½ green pepper
- 2 cans tuna, drained
- 12 black olives, pitted and sliced

Dressing:

- ⅔ cup olive oil
- ⅓ cup wine vinegar
- 2 cloves garlic, crushed
- 1 tablespoon Dijon mustard
- 1 tablespoon parsley flakes
- ½ teaspoon dried onion or onion powder
- 1 teaspoon Trocomare® (seasoned salt) or sea salt
- ¼ teaspoon pepper

Wash potatoes and boil unpeeled. Cook beans. Boil eggs. When they are done, drain and cool. While potatoes are cooking, mix ingredients for dressing in a jar with tight lid for shaking. Shake to mix.

When potatoes are cool, peel and cut into cubes and put in small bowl. Mince onion slice and add to potatoes. Drizzle with some of the dressing and let stand. Peel eggs and set aside in another bowl. Tear lettuce into separate salad bowl or large platter. Cut tomatoes into chunks and peppers into small squares. Sprinkle both over lettuce. Layer the marinated potatoes over the salad base. Then top with the green beans, the broken up tuna, the eggs cut in halves or quarters, and olive slices. Pour more dressing liberally over the whole salad and serve with the remaining dressing on the side.

Traditional Cole Slaw

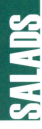
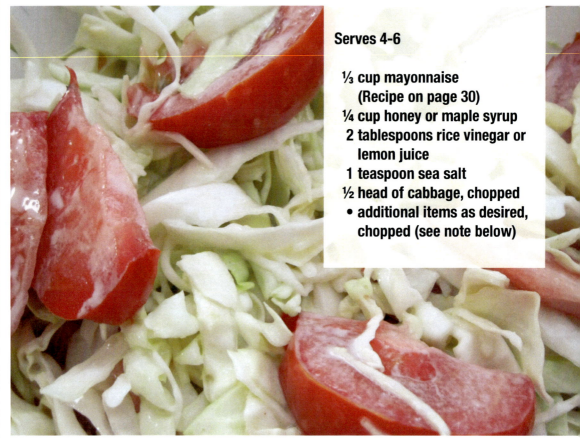

Serves 4-6

- ⅓ cup mayonnaise (Recipe on page 30)
- ¼ cup honey or maple syrup
- 2 tablespoons rice vinegar or lemon juice
- 1 teaspoon sea salt
- ½ head of cabbage, chopped
- additional items as desired, chopped (see note below)

Stir mayonnaise, sweetener, vinegar, and salt together in a small bowl or cup before stirring into salad of chopped cabbage and additional items.

Note: Traditional coleslaw can be varied by using shredded carrots, radishes, raisins, walnuts or pecans, canned pineapple, fresh tomatoes, zucchini, or sweet peppers along with cabbage. Use only one or two of the above items with the cabbage and the dressing.

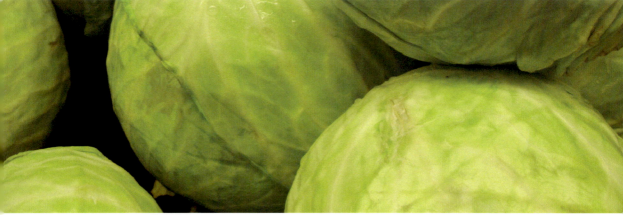

Spice of Life Specialty Foods PRESENTS

Zucchini Dulse Salad

Serves 4-6

- 3 cups zucchini, julienned
- 1 cup dulse, snipped
- ¼ cup olive oil
- 6 tablespoons rice vinegar
- 1 green onion, chopped
- 1 clove garlic, minced
- 1 teaspoon oregano
- 1 teaspoon basil
- 1 teaspoon parsley

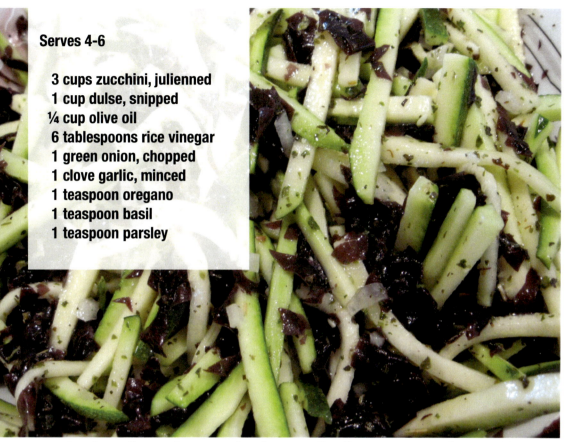

Combine all ingredients in a bowl. Mix well. Allow to marinate for several hours. This salad will keep a week in the refrigerator and the flavor improves with age.

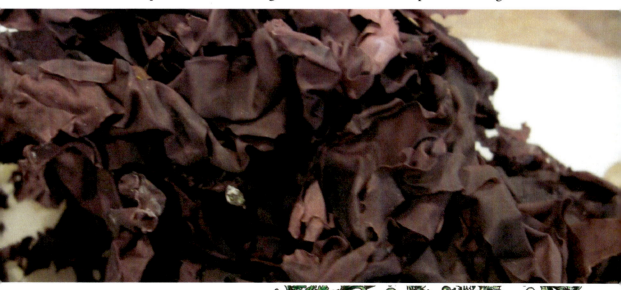

Wild Rice Salad

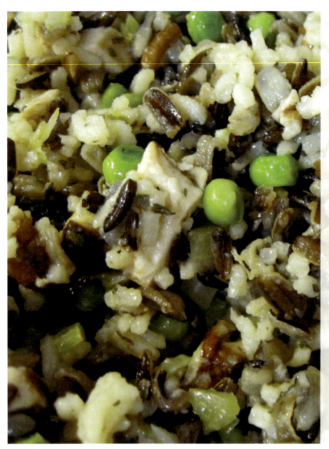

Serves 10-12

2 cups pecans
1 cup wild rice
4 cups water
2 teaspoons sea salt
1 cup white basmati rice
2 cups frozen peas
1 cup onions, chopped
1 cup celery, chopped
2 tablespoons olive oil
1 tablespoon basil
1 tablespoon Trocomare® (seasoned salt)
8 ounces chicken, grilled (or baked), cut into pieces
½ cup chicken broth (or broth from grilling chicken)
3 fresh tomatoes, cubed (optional)

Toast pecans in 300° oven for 18 minutes. Cool and break into small pieces. Set aside. Cook wild rice with water and salt in a pot on the stove top. Turn burner on high and bring to a boil. Then reduce heat to medium low and let simmer for 45-60 minutes until kernels are soft and fluffy. Add basmati rice. Stir occasionally for 15-20 minutes until fluffy and done. Add more water if needed. If you add more water, you will need to bring the rice back up to boiling and drop to simmer again. Add frozen peas. Pour into large bowl and stir. Set aside. Saute onions and celery in olive oil. Combine with peas and rice. Add basil and pecans. (Add optional tomatoes.) Sprinkle Trocomare® (seasoned salt) to taste. Add chicken and broth. Stir to mix. Add more salt if needed.

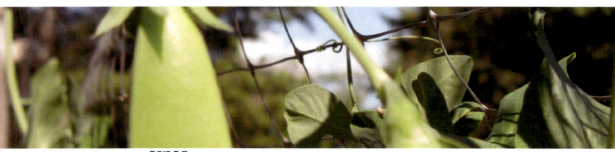

Spice of Life Specialty Foods PRESENTS

Rice Garbanzo Salad

Serves 4-6

- ½ cup onion, chopped
- ½ cup celery, chopped
- 2 tablespoons olive oil
- 1 cup frozen or fresh peas
- 2 cups garbanzo beans, cooked and drained
- 2 cups cooked rice
- 2 tablespoons fresh parsley, snipped
- ½ teaspoon basil
- 1 teaspoon vegetable bouillon paste or broth powder
- boiling water to dissolve bouillon
- 4 medium size tomatoes, cut in cubes
- 1 cup pecans, toasted and broken in pieces

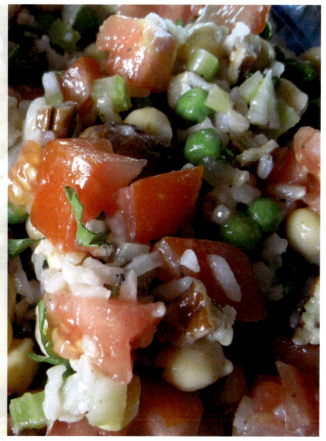

Sauté onion and celery in oil about five minutes. Add peas and cook five more minutes. Then combine sautéed vegetables with garbanzos, rice, parsley, and basil in a large salad bowl. In a small bowl, dissolve the bouillon in boiling water. Add to salad along with tomatoes and pecans. Toss to blend. Serve warm or at room temperature.

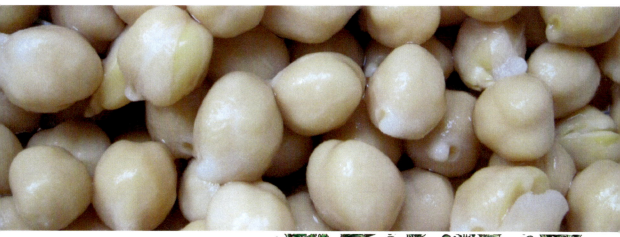

Potato Salad

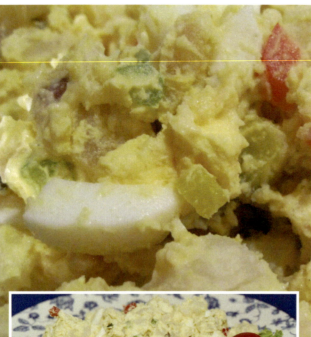

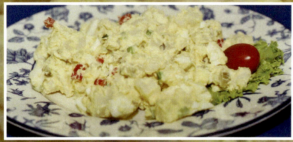

Makes 2 quarts

- 7 medium potatoes
- 7 eggs
- 1 slice onion, minced
- 1 stalk celery, minced
- 1 1-inch strip red pepper, minced
- 1 1-inch strip green pepper, minced
- 2 medium dill pickles, minced (or 3 small)
- ¼ cup mustard (or more as needed)
- ½ cup mayonnaise (or more as needed)
- ½ tablespoon Trocomare® (seasoned salt and more as needed)

Place potatoes in large pot. Add water to cover potatoes. Cook with pot covered on high to bring to a boil. Then drop temperature to medium-low. Cook for a total of 30-40 minutes or until potatoes are soft when pierced with fork

Place eggs in pot. Add water to cover eggs. Cook on high. Wait until eggs are at a rolling boil and set timer for 10 minutes. Drain hot water and add cold water. Continue until eggs are fairly cool. This makes it easier to peel eggs.

When potatoes are cooled, peel, chop, and put in large bowl. When eggs are cooled, peel, chop, and add to potatoes. Stir together and add onion, celery, red and green pepper, pickles, mustard, and mayonnaise. Mix well. Add Trocomare® (seasoned salt) to taste.

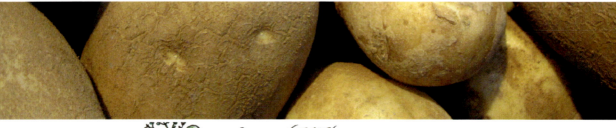

Spice of Life Specialty Foods **PRESENTS**

Tuna Noodle Salad

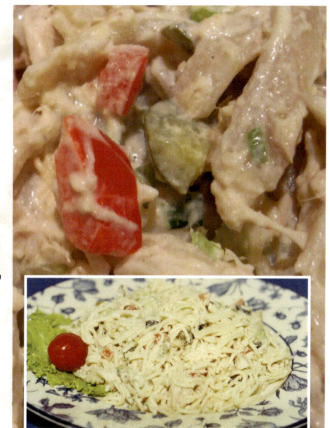

Makes about 7 servings

- water to boil noodles
- 4 servings noodles (thin spaghetti or whatever you prefer)
- 1 tablespoon sea salt
- 2 6-ounce cans tuna
- 1 stalk celery, chopped
- 2 green onions, chopped
- 1 1-inch strip of red pepper, chopped
- 1 1-inch strip of green pepper, chopped
- 2 dill pickles, chopped
- 10 black olives, chopped
- 2 teaspoons vegetable broth powder
- 1 cup mayonnaise
- 2 teaspoons Trocomare® (seasoned salt)

Bring water in a large pot to boil. Measure noodles for four servings into pot. Add the sea salt. Boil for ten minutes or until noodles are done. Drain noodles in colander and cool by running cold water over them. Continue to let noodles drain.

Drain cans of tuna and mix in a large bowl with chopped celery, onions, peppers, pickles, and olives. If using spaghetti noodles, cut shorter and mix into bowl with vegetable broth powder. Add mayonnaise and mix. Add Trocomare® and mix thoroughly.

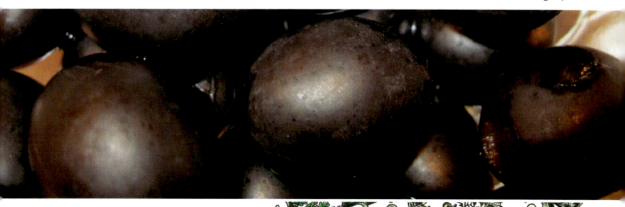

Common Sense Cooking

Mixed Bean Salad

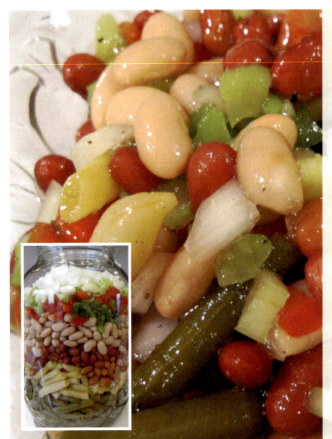

Makes large amount for potluck

The following can sizes are the regular size—about 2 cups or 1 pint.

- **4 cans 14.5-ounce regular cut green beans (or substitute a can of yellow wax beans for 1 can of green)**
- 1 can kidney beans
- 1 can pinto beans
- 1 can cannellini (white kidney) beans
- 1 can red beans
- 1 can great northern beans
- 1 1-inch slice sweet red pepper, finely chopped
- 1 1-inch slice sweet green pepper, finely chopped
- 1 cup celery (or 1 large stalk), finely chopped
- ½ cup red onion, finely chopped

Drain and rinse beans. Put in very large bowl or 1-gallon jar with lid (similar size to large pickle jars). Add vegetables: pepper, celery, and onion.

Mix the dressing in a large, glass measuring cup. Pour in the olive oil, vinegars, and honey. If the measuring cup is 3 cups or larger, you will not have to measure most of the dressing separately—just put the olive oil up to the ½ cup marking, add the apple cider vinegar to the 1 cup marking, and so on. Then add the Trocomare® and black pepper last. Mix lightly and pour dressing over beans. Mix loosely.

Let marinate for at least 3 hours before serving, mix before serving. If you use a large jar, you can simply turn the jar over to mix.

Dressing:
- ½ cup olive oil
- ½ cup apple cider vinegar
- ½ cup red wine vinegar
- 1½ cup honey
- 1 tablespoon + 1 teaspoon Trocomare® (seasoned salt)
- 1 teaspoon black pepper

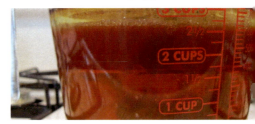

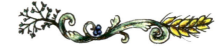

Spice of Life Specialty Foods PRESENTS

Three Bean Salad

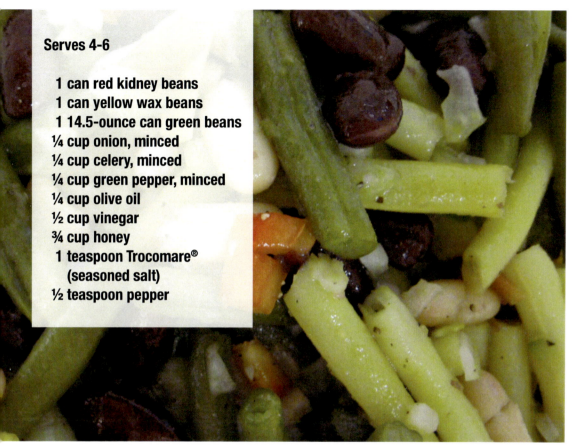

Serves 4-6

- 1 can red kidney beans
- 1 can yellow wax beans
- 1 14.5-ounce can green beans
- ¼ cup onion, minced
- ¼ cup celery, minced
- ¼ cup green pepper, minced
- ¼ cup olive oil
- ½ cup vinegar
- ¾ cup honey
- 1 teaspoon Trocomare® (seasoned salt)
- ½ teaspoon pepper

Rinse and drain kidney beans. Drain wax and green beans. Put in bowl. Add onion, celery, and green pepper. Mix dressing of olive oil, vinegar, honey, Trocomare® and pepper and pour over beans. Mix loosely and allow to marinate at least 3 hours before serving. Mix loosely before serving.

You can easily substitute beans in these salads. Try various combinations or replace another bean with lima beans.

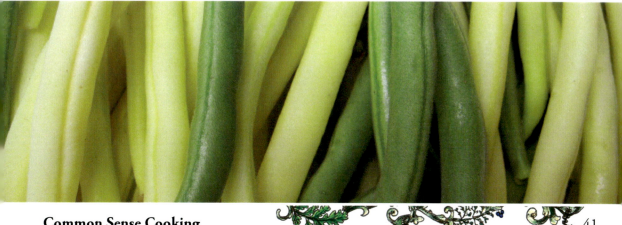

Beet-Herring Salad (Rosolli)

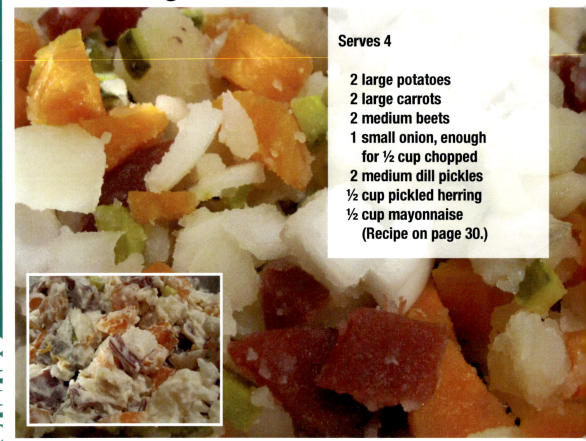

Serves 4

2 large potatoes
2 large carrots
2 medium beets
1 small onion, enough for ½ cup chopped
2 medium dill pickles
½ cup pickled herring
½ cup mayonnaise
(Recipe on page 30.)

For best flavor and nutritional value, boil the potatoes in their jackets. Also boil the carrots and the beets without peeling, but in separate kettles. After the vegetables are cooked, cool them in cold water and peel carefully. Cut into ½ inch cubes. Combine the carrots and potatoes in a bowl, but keep the beets out until last. Peel and mince the onion. Chop the dill pickles and herring, and add these along with the onion to carrots and potatoes. Just before serving, add the beets and toss to mix. Serve on a bed of green lettuce with mayonnaise as a dressing.

The mayonnaise may be mixed in or served on the side. This salad may be made without the herring or with hard boiled egg instead of the herring, or with pickled beets.

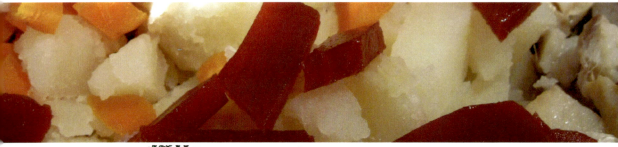

Spice of Life Specialty Foods PRESENTS

Cranberry Ring Salad

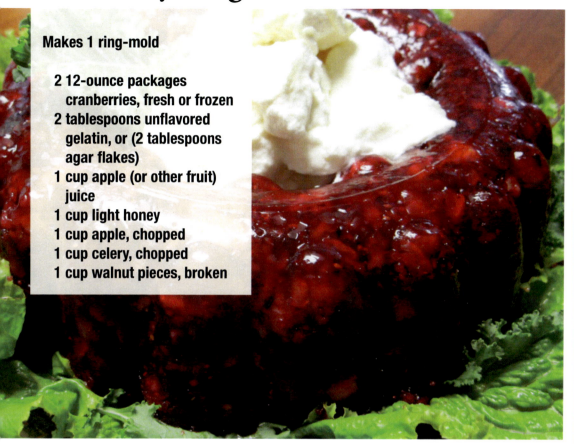

Makes 1 ring-mold

- 2 12-ounce packages cranberries, fresh or frozen
- 2 tablespoons unflavored gelatin, or (2 tablespoons agar flakes)
- 1 cup apple (or other fruit) juice
- 1 cup light honey
- 1 cup apple, chopped
- 1 cup celery, chopped
- 1 cup walnut pieces, broken

In a grinder or food processor, grind cranberries. (The food processor works best for frozen berries.) In a small saucepan over low heat, soften gelatin in apple juice, stirring until dissolved. If using agar agar, boil the agar with the juice for 5 minutes. Mix together cranberries, gelatin (or agar) and honey. Add apples, celery, and nuts. Mix well. Pour into a lightly oiled ring salad mold. This recipe fits perfectly into the three piece Tupperware® mold. Cover and refrigerate several hours or overnight until firm. Unmold onto a large plate that has a circle of fresh greens—leaf lettuce or parsley—around the edge. Fill the center with lightly sweetened whipped cream.

If using frozen berries, increase the gelatin to 3 envelopes and warm the honey with the gelatin and juice before adding to the cranberries.

Common Sense Cooking

Pam's Pepper Cheese Spread

Makes 1 pint

- 2 8-ounce boxes of cream cheese
- 1 clove of garlic, chopped or crushed
- 1 4-ounce can chili peppers, chopped
- 1 teaspoon oregano
- 6 large green olives, chopped (optional)

Mix all ingredients in a medium bowl. Allow flavors to blend before serving as a spread for whole grain crackers, bagels, or bread.

Original recipe is from Pam Niska.

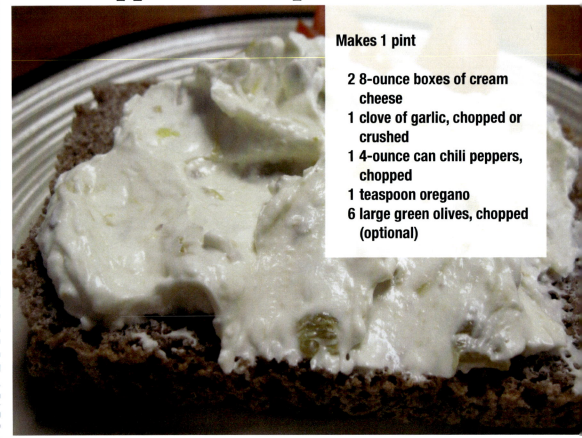

Chicken Salad Spread

Makes 4-5 pounds

- 3 slices red onion, minced
- 2-3 celery stalks, diced
- 2-3 dill pickles (5-6 tiny), diced
- ⅓ red pepper, diced
- 2 -2 ½ pounds cooked chicken, chopped
- • Trocomare® (seasoned salt)
- 2-3 cups mayonnaise

For smaller batch:
Makes 2 pounds

- 1 slice red onion, minced
- 1 large celery stalk, diced
- 1 large dill pickle, diced (or 2 small)
- 1 2-inch strip of sweet red pepper, diced
- 1 pound chopped chicken, cooked
- • Trocomare® (seasoned salt)
- 1 cup mayonnaise

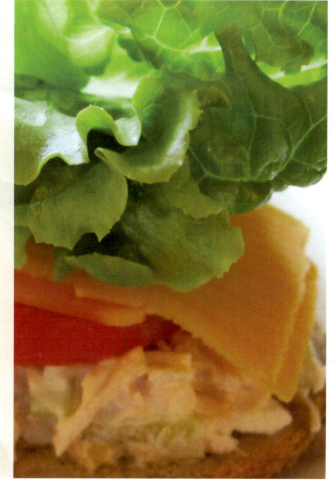

Dice all vegetables as small as possible. Cut up chicken and sprinkle with Trocomare® as you cut it. Mix chicken and vegetables in a bowl with mayonnaise. Add more mayonnaise and/or Trocomare® to taste.

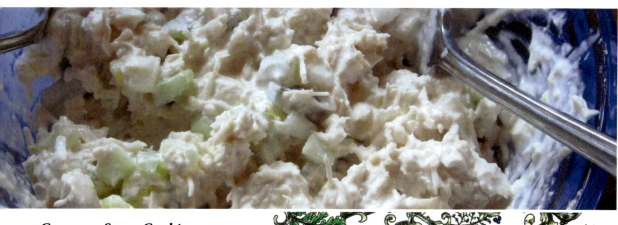

Tuna Salad Spread

SANDWICH SPREADS

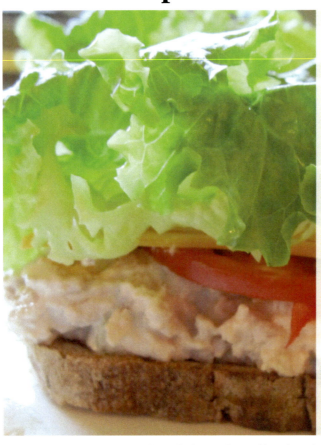

Makes 8-10 sandwiches

- 5 4.5-ounce cans tuna, drained (We prefer Starkist solid light tuna fillet in water.)
- 2 green onions, diced
- 1 celery stalk, diced (use one of inner stalks)
- 1 large dill pickle, diced (or 2 small or 5 tiny)
- ½ cup mayonnaise

For smaller batch:
Makes 2-4 sandwiches

- 2 cans tuna, drained
- 1 green onion, diced
- 1 medium celery stalk, diced
- 1 medium dill pickle, diced
- ¼ cup mayonnaise

Mix all ingredients well. A fork works well to break up tuna as you remove from can. Add more mayonnaise as desired.

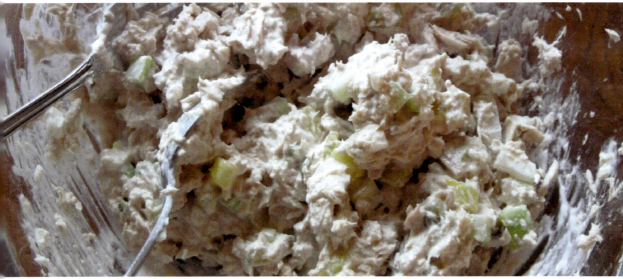

Spice of Life Specialty Foods PRESENTS

Egg Salad Spread

Makes 6-8 sandwiches

7-8 eggs
 1 green onion, diced
 1 tablespoon mustard
 2 tablespoons mayonnaise
 • Trocomare® (seasoned salt) to taste

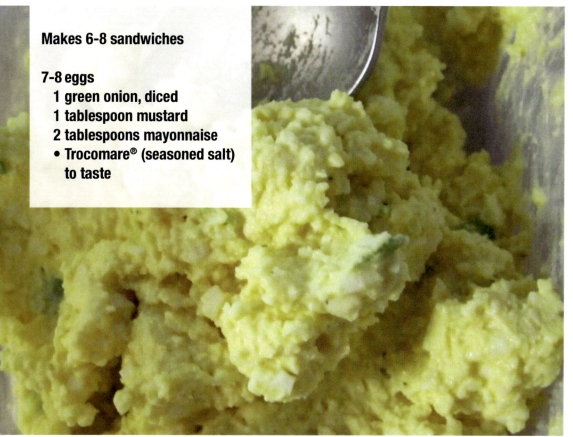

SANDWICH SPREADS

Put eggs in pot. Add water to cover eggs. Let eggs get to a rolling boil on high burner. Boil for 10 minutes. Cool eggs by running cold water into pan until pan and eggs are cool. Peel eggs. Put in bowl and mash using a potato masher. Add onions, mustard, mayonnaise, and a sprinkle of Trocomare®, and mix well. Add more mustard, mayonnaise or Trocomare® as desired.

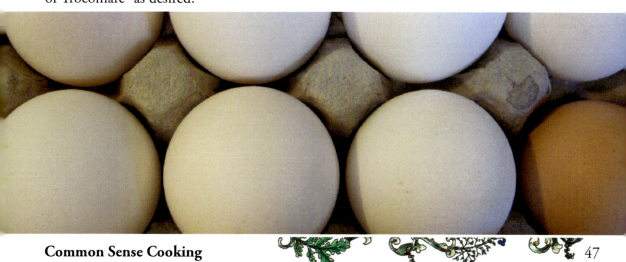

Common Sense Cooking

Hummus

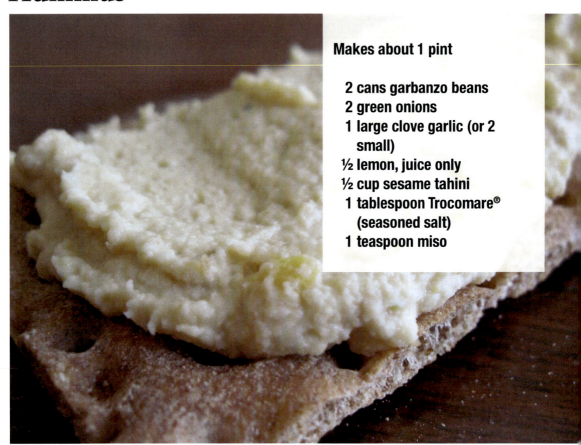

Makes about 1 pint

- 2 cans garbanzo beans
- 2 green onions
- 1 large clove garlic (or 2 small)
- ½ lemon, juice only
- ½ cup sesame tahini
- 1 tablespoon Trocomare® (seasoned salt)
- 1 teaspoon miso

Drain beans, saving liquid. Rinse onions and cut off roots and any bad parts. Peel garlic. Put all ingredients in a food processor. Puree until desired texture. Add back bean liquid as needed. May also be made using great northern beans.

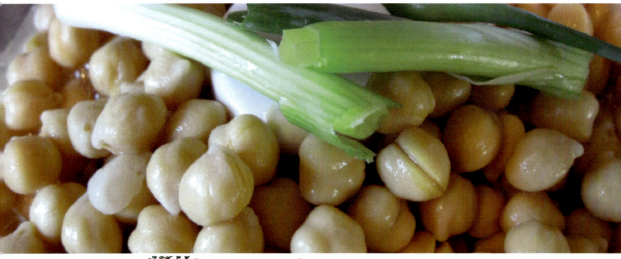

Granola

Makes 2½ pounds

  2 cups regular rolled oats
  2 cups quick oats
  ½ cup raw sunflower seeds
  ½ cup raw cashews
  1 cup almonds, sliced
  ½ cup olive oil
  ½ cup honey
  ½ cup maple syrup
  3 ounces raisins or dried cranberries (optional)

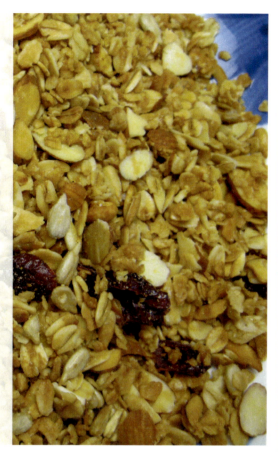

Preheat oven to 275°
Mix dry ingredients in large bowl: oats, sunflower seeds, cashews, and almonds. Add olive oil, honey, and maple syrup. Mix well. Put into lipped baking sheets or roaster pan. Bake for 2 ½ hours, stirring every 20-30 minutes until golden. When done, mix in the raisins. Cool.

Cinnamon Granola

  4 cups quick oats
  4 cups regular oats
  2 cups almonds, sliced
  1 cup pecans
  4 ounces oil
  4 ounces honey
  4 ounces maple syrup
  ½ teaspoon vanilla
  2 tablespoons cinnamon

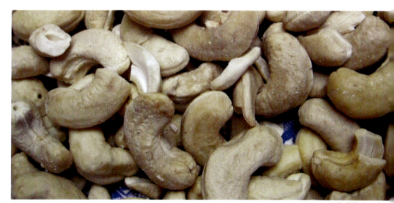

Preheat oven to 275°
Mix dry ingredients in large bowl: oats, almonds, and pecans. Add olive oil, honey, maple syrup, vanilla, and cinnamon. Mix well. Put into lipped baking sheets or roaster pan. Bake for 2 ½ hours, stirring every 20-30 minutes until golden. Cool.

Common Sense Cooking

Limppu Rye Bread

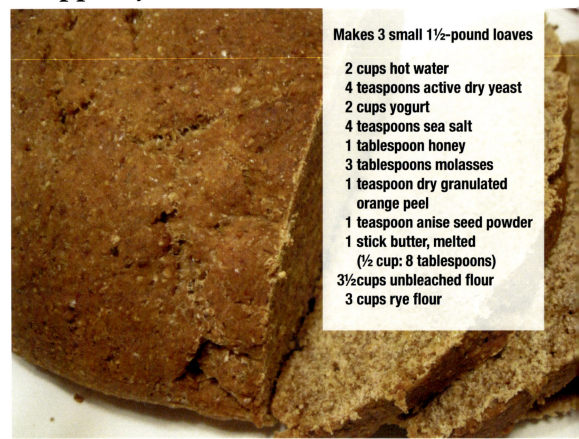

Makes 3 small 1½-pound loaves

2 cups hot water
4 teaspoons active dry yeast
2 cups yogurt
4 teaspoons sea salt
1 tablespoon honey
3 tablespoons molasses
1 teaspoon dry granulated orange peel
1 teaspoon anise seed powder
1 stick butter, melted
    (½ cup: 8 tablespoons)
3½ cups unbleached flour
3 cups rye flour

Pour hot water in mixing bowl. Add yeast and let sit for 5 minutes until foamy. Then stir in the yogurt, salt, honey, molasses, orange peel, anise seed, and butter. Add the flour ½ cup at a time and mix well. Place dough in greased bowl, cover with damp, warm cloth, and let rise in a warm place for one hour. Divide into thirds (about 1 ½ pounds each) and form into loaves. Place one loaf in each of three greased bread pans. Cover again and let rise for 45 minutes more. Bake in a 325° oven for 30 minutes.

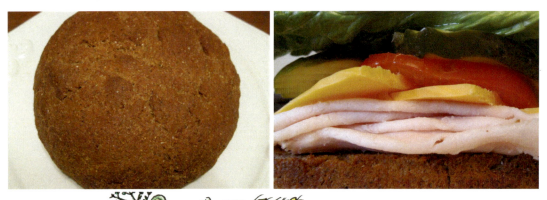

Finnish Sourdough Rye Bread

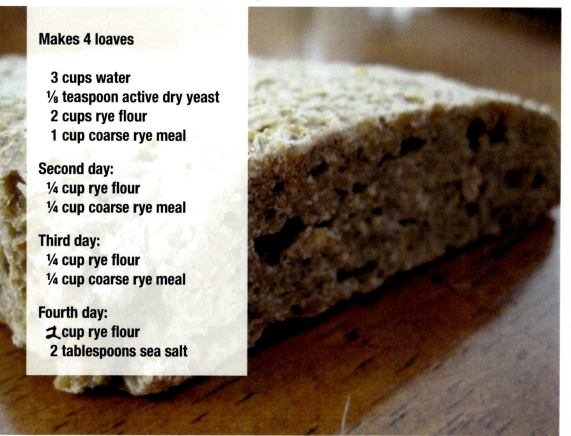

Makes 4 loaves

3 cups water
⅛ teaspoon active dry yeast
2 cups rye flour
1 cup coarse rye meal

Second day:
¼ cup rye flour
¼ cup coarse rye meal

Third day:
¼ cup rye flour
¼ cup coarse rye meal

Fourth day:
2 cup rye flour
2 tablespoons sea salt

In a large bowl, mix together water, yeast, and rye flour. Cover and let stand overnight. Next day, mix in rye flour. Cover again and let stand overnight. On third day, mix in rye flour. Cover again and let stand overnight. On fourth day add salt and flour and mix well.

Then divide dough into four equal parts on greased cookie sheets. With wet hands, pat the dough into four round loaves seven inches in diameter and a half inch high with a hole in the center. Put into a warm place to rise for 1-2 hours. Bake at 400° for 30 minutes. Dough may be formed into 2 round loaves in greased pie plates. Allow the same 2 hours for rising, but bake at 400° for an hour.

Wheat Bread

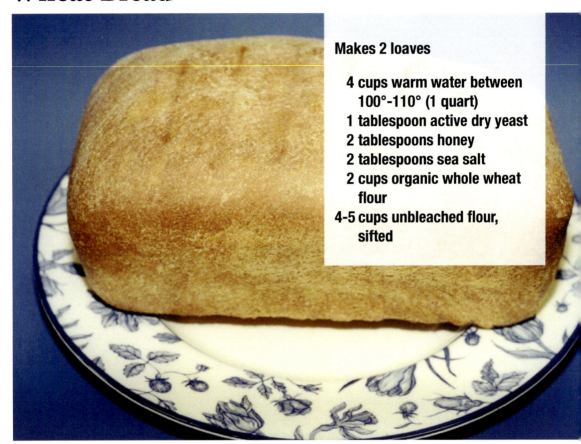

Makes 2 loaves

- 4 cups warm water between 100°-110° (1 quart)
- 1 tablespoon active dry yeast
- 2 tablespoons honey
- 2 tablespoons sea salt
- 2 cups organic whole wheat flour
- 4-5 cups unbleached flour, sifted

In a large bowl, put in water, yeast, honey and salt. Add the flour and mix until it forms a ball and pulls away from the sides of the bowl. If mixing by hand, the last mixing will be kneading on the counter.

Cover bowl, and put dough in a warm place to rise for one hour or until doubled in size. Butter two loaf pans. Form dough into loaves and put into greased pans. Prick loaves with a fork to get the air bubbles out. Cover and let rise again until double—about 20-25 minutes. Bake in a preheated, 425° oven for 30 minutes. (350° for a convection oven.)

The convection oven seals the outside crust and keeps the moisture in. In a regular oven the dough sometimes keeps rising as the bread bakes. If your mixer will only mix enough for one loaf, just cut the recipe in half.

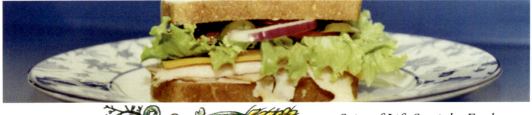

Spice of Life Specialty Foods PRESENTS

Multigrain Bread

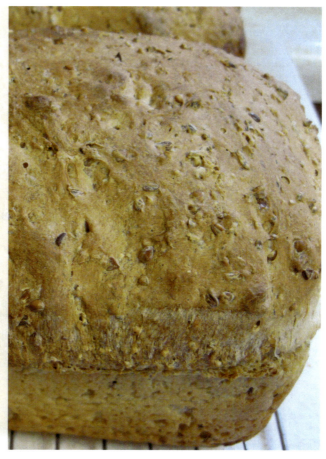

Makes 2 loaves

- ¼ cup millet
- ¼ cup buckwheat
- ¼ cup cracked barley
- ¼ cup cracked spelt
- ¼ cup cracked kamut
- ½ cup steel-cut oats
- 2 cups hot water (hot from tap will work)
- 2 cups warm water between 100°-110°
- 1 tablespoon active dry yeast
- 2 tablespoons honey
- 2 tablespoons sea salt
- 2 tablespoons flax seed
- 2 tablespoons sunflower seeds
- ¼ cup organic whole wheat flour
- 4-5 cups unbleached flour

The night before making bread, put millet, buckwheat, barley, spelt, kamut, and oats in a bowl or large jar and add the 2 cups of hot water. Cover with a lid and let sit overnight.

Add the soaked grains to the remaining 2 cups warm water, yeast, honey, salt, flax seed, sunflower seeds, and whole wheat flour. You can use a mixer. Then add unbleached flour and mix in until the dough forms a ball and pulls away from the sides of the bowl. This would include kneading by hand, if you are not using a mixer.

Cover bowl, and put dough in a warm place to rise for one hour or until doubled in size. Butter two loaf pans. Form dough into loaves and put into greased pans. Cover and let rise again until double—about 20-25 minutes. Bake in a preheated, 425° oven for 30 minutes. (350° for a convection oven.)

Whole Wheat Yeast Waffles

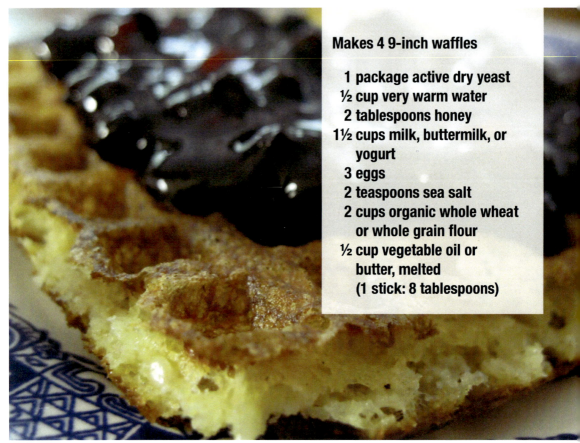

Makes 4 9-inch waffles

1 package active dry yeast
½ cup very warm water
2 tablespoons honey
1½ cups milk, buttermilk, or yogurt
3 eggs
2 teaspoons sea salt
2 cups organic whole wheat or whole grain flour
½ cup vegetable oil or butter, melted
(1 stick: 8 tablespoons)

    Soften the yeast in the water with the honey and allow to stand five minutes. Add remaining ingredients and mix well. Allow the batter to stand two or more hours to rise before baking. The batter can be mixed in the evening for baking the following morning. Bake on preheated hot waffle iron.

    Variations: Use one or several other whole grain flours to replace part or all of the wheat flour. Use soy milk or water instead of milk. Eggs may be omitted or replaced with egg substitute. Add ¼ cup of sesame seeds for added protein value.

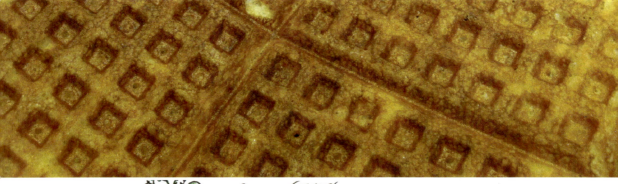

Gluten-Free Nisu

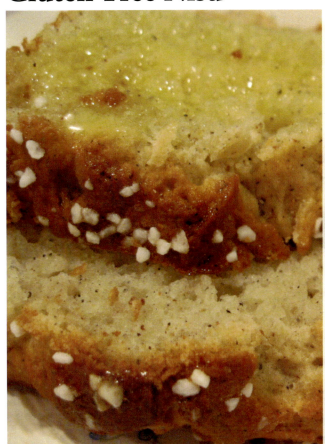

Makes two loaves

Based on Carl Keranen's gluten-free bread recipe.

- 1 tablespoon whole cardamom
- 3 large eggs
- 1 teaspoon cider vinegar
- ½ stick butter, melted
- 1 cup milk
- 1 cup hot water
- 1½ cup white rice flour
- ½ cup brown rice flour
- ½ cup potato starch
- ½ cup tapioca flour
- ½ cup arrowroot (or corn) starch
- 1 tablespoon xanthan gum
- ⅔ cup organic sugar
- 1 tablespoon sea salt
- 1 tablespoon baking yeast
- Swedish Pearl Sugar

Grind cardamom seeds in small spice or coffee grinder. Put eggs, vinegar, butter, milk, and hot water into bowl of mixer and beat with whisk until foamy. Add flours, starches, xanthan gum, sugar, salt, and yeast and mix in with paddle until smooth and thick. Dough will be more like brownies than bread. Divide into two buttered loaf pans and smooth down. Sprinkle with pearl sugar. Set in warm place to rise for about an hour or until doubled in bulk. This dough does not rise as quickly as bread dough. Bake at 400° for 35 minutes.

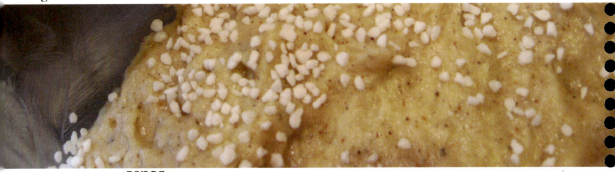

Spice of Life Specialty Foods PRESENTS

Caramel Corn

Serves 8

16 cups popcorn, popped
⅔ cup maple syrup
½ cup honey or rice syrup
½ cup unsalted butter
1 pinch of sea salt
2 teaspoons vanilla (optional)

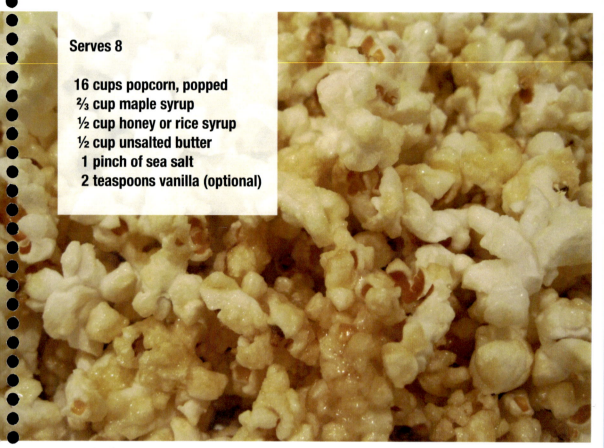

Preheat oven to 275°

Measure popcorn into large cake pans. Combine remaining ingredients in medium sized kettle. Stir over medium high heat until smooth and boiling. Boil about 5 minutes or until caramel reaches 235°. Pour over popcorn and mix to coat all kernels evenly. Bake at 275° for 20 minutes, stirring every 5 minutes. Cool and enjoy.

The caramel coating may also be used with plain dry cereals like puffed wheat or rice to make nutritious snacks.

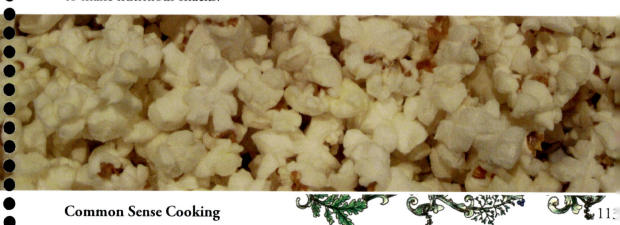

Gluten-free Gingerbread

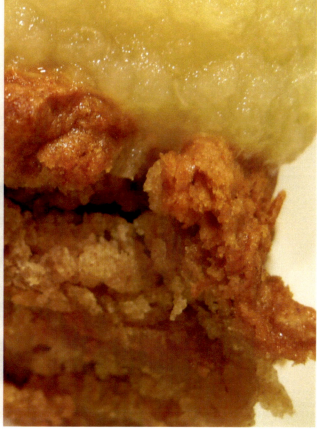

Makes 9-inch cake

- 1¼ cups rice flour (either white or brown or part of each)
- ¼ cup tapioca flour
- ¼ cup arrowroot starch
- ¼ cup potato starch
- 2 teaspoons xanthum gum
- ½ teaspoon cream of tartar
- 1 teaspoon sea salt
- 2 teaspoons baking powder
- 2 teaspoons baking soda
- 1½ teaspoons ground ginger
- 1 teaspoon cinnamon
- ¼ teaspoon ground cloves
- 1 cup maple syrup (or ½ cup each maple syrup and honey)
- 1 cup pureed or shredded, unpeeled zucchini (or applesauce)
- ½ cup butter, softened (1 stick: 8 tablespoons)

Preheat oven to 350.

Measure all ingredients into large bowl of electric mixer. Mix at medium speed until well blended, a few minutes. Pour into a greased 9" cake pan. Bake 30 - 40 minutes until cake springs back when touched lightly in the center. Serve warm topped with applesauce or lemon sauce and whipped cream.

Double ingredients for a 9 x 13 pan.

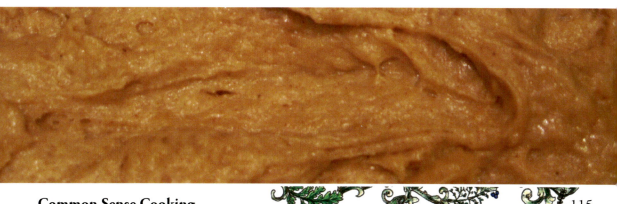

Common Sense Cooking

Index

A
agar agar 43
allspice 6, 19, 65, 69, 75
allspiced cider 19
almonds 49
anise 50, 105, 106
apple 43
apple cider 19, 40
Apple Pastry 111
applesauce 97, 115
apricot 14
arrowroot 11, 12, 14, 60, 77, 84, 93, 94, 95, 96, 114, 115

B
Baked Beans 29
Baked Cheesecake 83
baking powder 55, 56, 57, 61, 85, 89, 90, 97, 100, 101, 103, 104, 108, 111, 115
baking soda 57, 88, 97, 98, 99, 102, 104, 105, 109, 110, 115
balsamic vinegar 67, 68, 69
barley 26, 53, 56
bars. See **Chocolate Caramel Bars**; See also **Blueberry Bars**
basil 27, 28, 31, 35, 36, 37, 62, 64, 68, 71, 72, 73, 74, 81
basmati rice 36
Basting Sauce 67, 78.
   See **piirakka**; See **grilled fish or chicken**
Bavarian Cream Pie 92
bay leaf 21, 27, 64
beans 15, 22, 24, 28, 29, 33, 37, 40, 41, 48. See also **Baked Beans**; See also **cannellini**; See also **dark red kidney beans**; See also **garbanzo beans**; See also **great northern beans**; See also **green beans**; See also **kidney beans**; See also **pinto beans**; See also **red beans**; See also **red kidney beans**; See also **white kidney beans**; See also **white navy beans**
Bean Salad 40, 41
beef 27, 28, 62, 73, 80. See also **ground beef**
Beef Chili 28
Beef Meatballs 75
Beet-Herring Salad 42
beets 6, 42
berries 10, 12, 13, 43, 60, 84, 87, 92. See also **blueberries**; See also **blackberries**
Berry Sauce 11
blackberry jelly 13
black currant juice 69
blueberries 11, 56, 60, 93, 110
Blueberry Bars 110
Blueberry Muffins 56
Blueberry Pie Filling 93
Blue Cheese Salad Dressing 31
bouillon 16, 27, 37
bread 17, 18, 24, 25, 27, 44, 50, 52, 53, 59, 60, 74, 75, 76, 79, 114, 115. See also **Finnish Cardamom Bread**; See also **Finnish Sourdough Rye**; See also **Gluten-Free Gingerbread**; See also **Gluten-Free Pulla**; See also **Limppu Rye Bread**; See also **Multigrain Bread**; See also **Wheat Bread**; See also **Zucchini Bread**; See also **Zucchini Gingerbread**; See also **Cardamom Bread**
Bread and Butter Pickles 1
Bread Stuffing 17
broccoli 24
brown rice 18, 63, 78
brown rice flour 90, 114, 115
brown sugar 101, 103
buckwheat 16, 53, 56
buckwheat kasha 16
buns 58, 60. See also **Cinnamon Buns**; See also **Fruit & Nut Filled Buns**
Butter Biscuits 83, 86, 92
buttermilk 54, 55, 56, 57
butterscotch 109, 112

C
cabbage 7, 26, 34
cake 59, 72, 84, 85, 88, 97, 113. See also **Baked Cheesecake**; See also **Carrot Cake**; See also **Fruit Cake**; See also **Raspberry-Filled Cake**; See also **Zucchini Gingerbread**; See also **No-Bake Strawberry Cheesecake**
calcium phosphate 12, 13, 14
candy 112. See also **Caramel Corn**; See also **Chocolate Truffle**
cannellini 40
caramel 109, 113
Caramel Corn 113
cardamom 58, 59, 60, 100, 101, 105, 114
Cardamom Bread 58, 114
Cardamom White Caps 101
carrot 18, 20, 24, 26
Carrot Cake 88
cashews 49
casserole 21, 29, 63
cauliflower 5, 24
cayenne pepper 2
celery 1, 2, 5, 17, 18, 22, 23, 24, 27, 28, 32, 36, 37, 38, 39, 40, 41, 43, 45, 46, 63, 64, 72, 76, 80
Celery Chow Chow 5
celery seed 1, 2, 5, 32
cereal. See **Cinnamon Granola**; See also **Granola**
cheddar cheese 72
cheese 21, 31, 32, 44, 73, 79, 81, 83, 86, 88, 104. See also **soy cheese**; See also **ricotta**
cheesecake. See **Baked Cheesecake**; See also **No-Bake Strawberry Cheesecake**
cherries 89
chicken 16, 22, 23, 36, 45, 67, 68. See also **Grilled Chicken**; See also **Grilled Fish or Chicken**
chicken broth 16, 22, 23, 36
Chicken Noodle Soup 23
Chicken Salad Spread 45
Chicken Vegetable Soup 22
chili. See **Beef Chili**
chili peppers 44
chili powder 28, 73
Chocolate Caramel Bars 109
Chocolate Chip Cookies 98, 99
chocolate chips 98, 99, 106, 108, 109, 112
   white chocolate chips 99
Chocolate Truffle 112
chokecherries 13
cider
   allspiced 19
   cider vinegar 2, 5, 9, 19, 30, 32, 40, 67, 114
cilantro 9
cinnamon 6, 10, 19, 20, 49, 57, 58, 59, 61, 65, 69, 88, 91, 94, 97, 98, 102, 103, 104, 105, 108, 110, 111, 115
Cinnamon Buns 59
Cinnamon Granola 49
cinnamon rolls 58, 61
cinnamon sticks 6, 10
citron 105
cloves 3, 4, 8, 9, 17, 22, 32, 33, 57, 62, 69, 70, 72, 73, 77, 91, 97, 102, 104, 105, 115
coconut 74, 106, 108
Cole Slaw 34
cookies. See **Cardamom White Caps**; See also **Chocolate Chip Cookies**; See also **Cranberry White Chocolate Chip Cookies**; See also **Finnish Cardamom Cookies**; See also **Finnish Ginger Cookies**; See also **German Peppernuts**;
   See also **Ginger Snaps**;
   See also **Granola Chews**;
   See also **Macaroons**; See also **Pumpkin Cookies**
coriander 75
corn 24, 27
cornstarch 85, 86, 87, 94, 96, 110, 114
counter top dill pickles 4. See also **fermented**
crab 72
cracked barley 53
cracked kamut 53
cracked spelt 53
cracker crumbs 74
cranberries 10, 43, 49, 89, 99
Cranberry Ring Salad 43
Cranberry Sauce 10
Cranberry White Chocolate Chip Cookies 99
cream 5, 11, 31, 43, 75, 85, 90, 91, 92, 95, 97, 100, 103, 106, 112
cream cheese 32, 44, 72, 83, 86, 88, 104
Cream Cheese Salad Dressing 32
cream of tartar 115
crushed red pepper 29, 65, 72, 76, 77
crust
   pie crust 52, 60, 78, 80, 81, 82, 83, 84, 90, 91, 93, 94, 110
cucumber 1, 2, 3, 4, 5
currant 13, 69

D
dark red kidney beans 28
dates 89
di-calcium phosphate 12, 13
Dijon mustard 33
dill 3, 4, 38, 42, 45, 46
Dill Pickles 3, 4
dill pickles 38, 39, 42, 45
drink. See **Allspiced Cider**
   cider 19
dulse 35

E
egg 16, 42, 56, 60, 67, 74, 75, 76, 96, 100, 102, 106
eggs 30, 33, 38, 47, 54, 55, 57, 58, 71, 73, 79, 80, 82, 83, 84, 85, 88, 89, 91, 99, 101, 104, 105, 107, 114
Egg Salad Spread 47
egg whites 106

F
fennel 62, 73, 81
fermented 4
filling. See **Fruit Filling**; See also **Honey Walnut Filling**
Finnish Cardamom Bread 58
Finnish Cardamom Cookies 100
Finnish Ginger Cookies 103

Finnish Karelian Pastries. See **Karjalan Piirakkas**
Finnish Sourdough Rye 51
fish 15, 30, 67, 70, 74. See also **Fish Fillets in Tomato Sauce**; See also **Fried Fish**; See also **Grilled Fish**; See also **Grilled Fish or Chicken**; See also **herring**
Fish Fillets in Tomato Sauce 70
flax seed 53
French Garden Salad 33
Fried Fish 74
frosting 88, 104, 106
Fruit & Nut Filled Buns 60
Fruit Cake 89
Fruit Filling 60

G
garbanzo beans 37, 48
Garbanzo Salad 37
garlic 3, 4, 8, 9, 17, 18, 22, 23, 24, 28, 31, 32, 33, 35, 44, 48, 62, 63, 64, 65, 69, 70, 72, 73, 74, 75, 76, 77, 80
gelatin 43, 84, 92
German Peppernuts 105
Ghiradelli 99
ginger 29, 69, 91, 97, 102, 103, 104, 115
Ginger Snaps 102
gluten-free 90, 114, 115
Gluten-Free Gingerbread 115
Gluten-Free Pulla (Nisu) 114
Gluten-Free Pie Crust 90
graham crackers 84
grain 26, 53, 56. See also **barley**; See also **buckwheat**; See also **kamut**; See also **oats**; See also **rye**; See also **spelt**; See also **wheat**
Granola 49, 108. See also **Cinnamon Granola**
Granola Chews 108
grapefruit 10, 69
great northern beans 40, 48
green beans 22, 24, 33, 40, 41
green olives 44
green onion 20, 26, 31, 35, 46, 47
green pepper 9, 28, 33, 38, 39, 40, 41, 81
green split peas 25
Grilled Chicken Marinades 68
Grilled Fish or Chicken 67
Grilled Turkey 65
Grilled Whole Turkey 66
groats 16
ground beef 28, 62, 73, 80
guar gum 90

H
half and half 21, 75, 77, 91, 106
herring 42
Honey Walnut Filling 60

Hummus 48
Hunter's Stew 27

I
Italian sausage 73, 81
Italian Style Salad Dressing 31

J
jalapeños 9
jam. See also **low/alternate sugar jam**; See also **Pepperidge Farm Style Apricot Jam**
jelly 12, 13. See also **Currant Jelly**; See also **Wild Blackberry Jelly**; See also **Low/Alternate Sugar Jam or Jelly**
juice 7, 9, 12, 13, 19, 22, 28, 31, 34, 43, 48, 56, 64, 65, 67, 68, 69, 70, 83, 92, 94, 96

K
kamut 53, 56
Karelian Pastries. See **Karjalan Piirakkas**
Karjalan Piirakkas 78
kasha. See **Buckwheat Kasha**
ketchup 29
kidney beans 28, 40, 41
kombu 24, 29
kuzu 12, 77

L
Lamb or Beef Meatballs 75
Lamb Roast 64
Lasagna 72, 73. See also **Seafood Lasagna**
leaf lettuce 33, 43
Leibniz Butter Biscuits 83, 86, 92
lemon 19, 48, 65, 69, 74, 83, 97
Lemon Herb Marinade 68
lemon juice 9, 31, 34, 67, 70, 92, 94, 96
lemon zest 96
lime 69
Limppu Rye Bread 50
LM pectin 12
low-methoxyl pectin. See **LM pectin**
Low/Alternate Sugar Jam or Jelly 12

M
Macaroons 106
maple sugar 59, 61, 85, 86, 94, 101, 104, 110
marinade 64, 65, 67, 68, 69. See also **Lemon Herb Marinade**; See also **Spicy Marinade**; See also **Teriyaki Marinade**; See also **Grilled Fish or Chicken**
Marinade for Grilled Turkey 65
Marinade for Lamb Roast 64

marjoram 17, 24, 69, 71, 72, 74, 77, 81
mayonnaise 30, 31, 34, 38, 39, 42, 45, 46, 47
meatballs. See **Turkey Meatballs**; See also **Lamb or Beef Meatballs**
milk 21, 32, 54, 55, 56, 57, 58, 61, 72, 76, 77, 78, 79, 82, 84, 91, 101, 105, 111, 114
millet 15, 53, 56
millet flour 90
miso 25, 48
Miso Soup 26
Mixed Bean Salad 40
molasses 50, 102
mozzarella 73, 81
Mrs. Richardson's Butterscotch Caramel 109
muffins. See **Whole Wheat Blueberry Muffins**
Multigrain Bread 53
mushroom 26, 76, 81
mushrooms 16, 63, 72, 77
Mushroom Sauce 77
mushroom sauce 72
mustard 5, 29, 30, 32, 33, 38, 47, 75
mustard seed 1, 2

N
Naturally fermented 4
Nisu 58. See also **Finnish Cardamom Bread**
No-Bake Strawberry Cheesecake 84
noodles 23, 27, 39, 62, 72, 73
nori 20
Nori Rolls 20
nutmeg 65, 69, 82, 91, 104, 105, 108
nuts. See **almonds**; See also **cashews**; See also **pecans**; See also **sunflower seeds**; See also **walnuts**

O
oats 49, 53, 98, 99, 108, 109, 110
Olive Oil Pickles 2
olives
  black 33, 39, 81
  green olives 44
onion 1, 2, 9, 15, 18, 20, 22, 23, 24, 25, 26, 27, 28, 31, 32, 33, 35, 37, 38, 40, 41, 42, 45, 46, 47, 62, 63, 64, 65, 69, 71, 72, 73, 74, 75, 76, 77, 80, 81
onion powder 33, 64, 69, 74
orange 10, 69
orange juice 19
orange peel 50, 105
oregano 9, 17, 24, 31, 35, 44, 62, 64, 68, 74, 81

organic sugar 6, 58, 61, 83, 85, 86, 87, 89, 92, 93, 99, 100, 102, 104, 108, 109, 111, 114

P
pancakes. See **Whole Wheat Pancakes**; See also **Potato Pancakes**
paprika 63, 72, 74, 77
Parmesan 31, 73
parsley 17, 21, 23, 24, 28, 31, 33, 35, 37, 43, 62, 63, 68, 72, 73, 74, 76, 77, 81
pastry. See **Apple Pastry**
Pasty 80
pearl sugar 58, 114
peas 24, 25, 27, 36, 37
pecans 34, 36, 37, 49, 60, 89, 107
Pecan Tarts 107
pectin 12, 13, 14
pepper. See **chili peppers**; See also **green pepper**
Pepper Cheese Spread 44
Pepperidge Farm Style Apricot Jam 14
peppermint 112
peppernuts. See **German Peppernuts**
pickle 20, 40, 45, 46
Pickled Beets 6
pickles 1, 2, 3, 4. See also **Bread and Butter Pickles**; See also **Celery Chow Chow**; See also **Olive Oil Pickles**; See also **Pickled Beets**; See also **Dill Pickles**; See also **Sauerkraut**
pie. See **Bavarian Cream Pie**; See also **Blueberry Pie Filling**; See also **Pumpkin Pie**; See also **Raspberry Cream Pie**; See also **Rhubarb Custard Pie**; See also **Zucchini Pie**
Pie Crust 90
piirakkas. See **Karjalan Piirakkas**
pineapple 34, 89
pinto beans 40
pizza 60, 81
Pomona's Universal Pectin 12
popcorn 113
potatoes 21, 22, 24, 27, 33, 38, 42, 71, 76, 80. See also **Scalloped Potatoes**
Potato Pancakes 71
Potato Salad 38
potato starch 114, 115
poultry seasoning 17, 18, 22, 23, 24, 67, 76
powdered sugar 61, 101, 104, 105, 111
Pulla 58

pumpkin 91, 104
Pumpkin Cookies 104
Pumpkin Pie 91

Q
quinoa flour 90

R
raisins 34, 49, 57, 89, 104
raspberries 11, 60, 85, 86, 87, 92
Raspberry-Filled Cake 85, 86
Raspberry Cream Pie 86
Raspberry Sauce 85, 86, 87
red beans 40
red kidney beans 28, 41
red onion 40, 45
red pepper 9, 17, 21, 22, 24, 29, 31, 32, 33, 38, 39, 40, 45, 62, 64, 65, 68, 69, 72, 76, 77
red wine 30, 32, 40, 62, 67, 68, 69
rhubarb 60, 82
Rhubarb Custard Pie 82
rice 18, 20, 34, 35, 36, 37, 63, 70, 74, 76, 77, 78, 79, 113. *See also* **basmati rice**; *See also* **brown rice**; *See also* **wild rice**
rice flour 90, 114, 115
Rice Garbanzo Salad 37
Rice Stuffing 18
rice syrup 113
rice vinegar 34, 35, 70
rice yield 18
ricotta 73
roast. *See* **Lamb Roast**; *See also* **turkey roast**
rolls. *See* **cinnamon rolls**
romaine 33
Romano 73
Rose Hip Sauce 95
rosemary 17, 24, 62, 64, 69, 74
Rosolli. *See* **Beet-Herring Salad**
rum 89, 99, 112
rye bread 25. *See also* **Limppu Rye Bread**; *See also* **Finnish Sourdough Rye**
rye flour 50, 51, 78

S
sage 17, 24, 62, 64, 65, 69, 74
salad 28, 30, 31, 32, 33, 34, 35, 36, 37, 42, 43. *See also* **Cranberry Ring Salad**; *See also* **French Garden Salad**; *See also* **Garbanzo Salad**; *See also* **Mixed Bean Salad**; *See also* **Potato Salad**; *See also* **Rice Garbanzo Salad**; *See also* **Beet-Herring Salad**; *See also* **Cole Slaw**; *See also* **Three Bean Salad**; *See also* **Tuna Noodle Salad**; *See also* **Wild Rice Salad**; *See also* **Zucchini Dulse Salad**
salad dressing. *See* **Cream Cheese Salad Dressing**; *See also* **Italian Style Salad Dressing**; *See also* **Blue Cheese Salad Dressing**
Salade Niçoise. *See* **French Garden Salad**
salad oil 30, 31, 32
salsa. *See* **Victoria's Salsa**
sandwich spread. *See* **Egg Salad Spread**; *See also* **Hummus**; *See also* **Pepper Cheese Spread**; *See also* **Tuna Salad Spread**; *See also* **Chicken Salad Spread**
sauce. *See* **Mushroom Sauce**; *See also* **Raspberry Sauce**; *See also* **Rose Hip Sauce**; *See also* **marinade**; *See also* **Tomato Sauce**; *See also* **Zucchini Lemon Sauce**; *See also* **Cranberry Sauce**; *See also* **Berry Sauce**
Sauerkraut 7
sausage 73, 81
savory 17, 24, 62, 64, 69, 72, 74, 77, 81
Scalloped Potatoes 21
Seafood Lasagna 72
sesame oil 26
sesame seeds 54
sesame tahini 48
shiitake mushroom 26
shrimp 72
soup 22, 24, 25, 26. *See also* **Chicken Noodle Soup**; *See also* **Hunter's Stew**; *See also* **Miso Soup**; *See also* **Split Pea Soup**; *See also* **Turkey Soup**; *See also* **Chicken Vegetable Soup**; *See also* **Beef Chili**
Sourdough Rye Bread 51
soy cheese 72
soymage sour cream 72
soy milk 54, 55, 56, 72
soy sauce 64, 65, 69, 72, 77
spaghetti 39, 62
spelt 53, 56
spice chart vi
Spicy Marinade 69
split peas 25
Split Pea Soup 25
squash 91, 104
Starkist 46
steel-cut oats 53
stew. *See* **Hunter's Stew**
strawberries 60, 84, 92
Strawberry Cheesecake 84
stuffing. *See* **Rice Stuffing**; *See also* **Bread Stuffing**
sugar. *See* **brown sugar**; *See also* **turbinado sugar**; *See also* **maple sugar**; *See also* **organic sugar**; *See also* **powdered sugar**
sunflower seeds 49, 53
sushi. *See* **Nori Rolls**
sweetener. *See* **rice syrup**; *See also* **honey**; *See also* **maple syrup**; *See also* **organic sugar**; *See also* **maple sugar**; *See also* **brown sugar**; *See also* **turbinado sugar**; *See also* **powdered sugar**

T
tacos 28
tahini 48
tamari 64, 65, 69, 72, 77
tangerines 10
tapioca 5, 72, 93
tapioca flour 90, 115
tarts. *See* **Pecan Tarts**; *See also* **Granola Chews**
temperatures baking/cooking v
Teriyaki Marinade 69
Three Bean Salad 41
thyme 17, 24, 25, 62, 64, 65, 69, 70, 71, 74, 77
tomatoes 8, 9, 27, 33, 34, 36, 37
tomato juice 70
Tomato Sauce 8, 70
Trocomare* v
truffle. *See* **Chocolate Truffle**
tuna 33, 39, 46
Tuna Noodle Salad 39
Tuna Salad Spread 46
turbinado sugar 101
turkey 16, 17, 18, 24, 28, 63, 65, 66, 76, 81. *See also* **Grilled Turkey**; *See also* **turkey roast**
turkey broth 24, 63
turkey fat 24
turkey Italian sausage 81
Turkey Meatballs 76
Turkey Rice Casserole 63
turkey roast 18
Turkey Soup 24
turmeric 5

U
umeboshi paste 20

V
vanilla 11, 49, 57, 60, 61, 83, 84, 85, 86, 87, 88, 89, 92, 95, 98, 101, 104, 107, 110, 111, 113
vegetable broth powder 18, 36, 39
venison 27
Victoria's Salsa 9

W
waffles 11, 54, 87. *See also* **Whole Wheat Yeast Waffles**
wakame 25, 26
walnut 43, 89
walnuts 34, 60, 101, 104, 105
wheat 5, 18, 52, 53, 54, 55, 56, 62, 88, 113
Wheat Bread 52
whipping cream 85, 86, 90, 92, 103
white chocolate chips 99
white kidney beans 40
white navy beans 29
white rice flour 114, 115
whole turkey 66
Whole Wheat Blueberry Muffins 56
whole wheat flour 52, 53, 55, 56
Whole Wheat Pancakes 55
whole wheat pastry flour 88
Whole Wheat Yeast Waffles 54
Wild Blackberry Jelly 13
wild rice 18, 36
Wild Rice Salad 36
wine 30, 32, 33, 40, 62, 64, 67, 68, 69

X
xanthan gum 90, 114, 115

Y
yeast 50, 51, 52, 53, 54, 58, 81, 114
yellow wax beans 40, 41
yogurt 31, 32, 50, 54, 55, 56, 57, 61, 84

Z
zucchini 34, 35, 57, 71, 94, 95, 96, 97, 115
Zucchini Bread 57
Zucchini Dulse Salad 35
Zucchini Gingerbread 97
zucchini gingerbread 95, 96, 115
Zucchini Lemon Sauce 96
Zucchini Pie 94

Spice of Life Specialty Foods PRESENTS

Whole Wheat Blueberry Muffins

Makes 1 dozen muffins

- 2 cups organic whole wheat flour
- 4 teaspoons baking powder
- ½ teaspoon sea salt
- 1 cup wild blueberries, fresh or frozen
- ¾ cup milk, buttermilk, yogurt or soy milk
- ½–⅔ cup honey or maple syrup
- 1 egg, beaten
- 4 tablespoons butter, melted (½ stick: ¼ cup) or 3 tablespoons oil

Preheat oven to 425°

Melt the butter as the oven preheats.

Measure the flour into a large mixing bowl. Add baking powder, salt, and blueberries. Mix well. Put remaining ingredients into food processor or blender and blend until mixed. Then add to dry ingredients. Mix until just blended. Fill lined or lightly greased muffin tins two-thirds full. Bake for 25 minutes.

Variations: Soy milk or water may be used in place of the milk. Honey or concentrated fruit juice may be used in place of the maple syrup. The egg can be eliminated or exchanged for egg replacer. Use one or a combination of other whole grain flours like barley, oat, buckwheat, millet, spelt, or kamut.

Marinade for Grilled Turkey

Makes 1 pint

- 1 medium onion
- 1 clove garlic
- ¼ cup tamari/soy sauce
- ¼ cup olive oil
- 1 tablespoon honey or maple syrup
- 1 teaspoon black pepper
- 1 teaspoon crushed red pepper
- ½ teaspoon cinnamon
- ½ teaspoon nutmeg
- 2 teaspoons dried sage
- 2 teaspoons dried thyme
- 1 teaspoon ground allspice
- 2 teaspoons Trocomare® (seasoned salt) or sea salt
- 1 lemon, juice only

Blend all ingredients in blender. Coat about 3 pounds of turkey steaks or cubes, and allow to marinate several hours or overnight before grilling. Use 1½ pounds of turkey for half recipe of marinade or 3 pounds for full recipe.

Multigrain Bread

Makes 2 loaves

- ⅓ cup millet
- ⅓ cup buckwheat
- ¾ cup cracked barley
- ¾ cup cracked spelt
- ¾ cup cracked kamut
- ¾ cup steel-cut oats
- 2 cups hot water (hot from tap will work)
- 2 cups warm water between 100°-110°
- 1 tablespoon active dry yeast
- 4 tablespoons honey
- 2 tablespoons sea salt
- 2 tablespoons flax seed
- 2 tablespoons sunflower seeds
- 4-5 cups unbleached flour

The night before making bread, put millet, buckwheat, barley, spelt, kamut, and oats in a bowl or large jar and add the 2 cups of hot water. Cover with a lid and let sit overnight.

Add the soaked grains to the remaining 2 cups warm water, yeast, honey, salt, flax seed, sunflower seeds, and whole wheat flour. You can use a mixer. Then add unbleached flour and mix in until the dough forms a ball and pulls away from the sides of the bowl. This would include kneading by hand, if you are not using a mixer.

Cover bowl, and put dough in a warm place to rise for one hour or until doubled in size. Butter two loaf pans. Form dough into loaves and put into greased pans. Cover and let rise again until double—about 20-25 minutes. Bake in a preheated, 425° oven for 30 minutes. (350° for a convection oven.)

CORRECTIONS

Whole Wheat Pancakes

Makes 12 5-inch pancakes

- 2 cups organic whole wheat flour
- 1 teaspoon sea salt
- 2 teaspoons baking powder
- 1½ cups milk, buttermilk, or yogurt
- 2 eggs
- 2 tablespoons oil or butter, melted

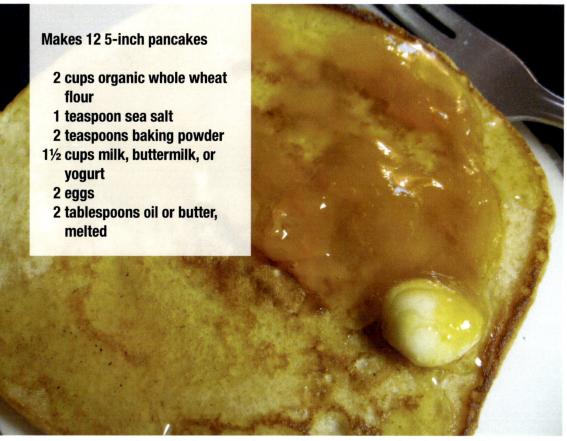

Stir flour, salt, and baking powder together in a mixing bowl. Add milk, eggs, and oil. Stir to mix ingredients. Spoon onto hot griddle. Turn after a couple minutes to cook other side.

Variations: Use one or several other whole grain flours to replace all or part of the wheat flour. Use soy milk or water in place of the milk. Eggs may be omitted or replaced with a egg substitute.

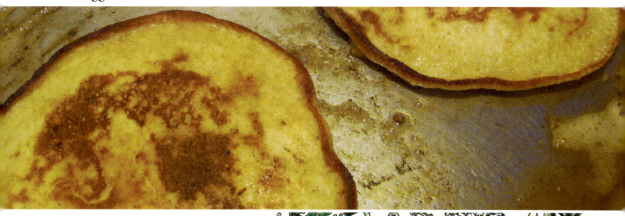

Whole Wheat Blueberry Muffins

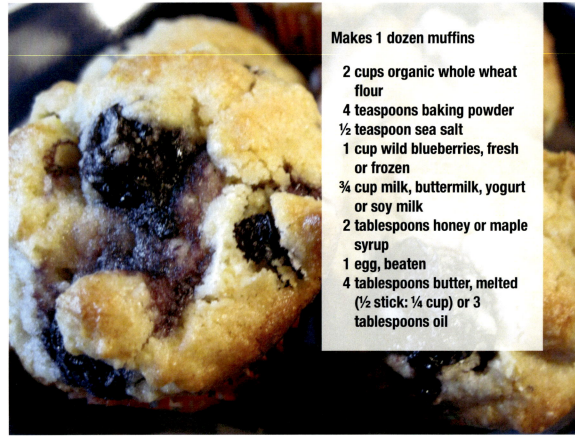

Makes 1 dozen muffins

- 2 cups organic whole wheat flour
- 4 teaspoons baking powder
- ½ teaspoon sea salt
- 1 cup wild blueberries, fresh or frozen
- ¾ cup milk, buttermilk, yogurt or soy milk
- 2 tablespoons honey or maple syrup
- 1 egg, beaten
- 4 tablespoons butter, melted (½ stick: ¼ cup) or 3 tablespoons oil

Preheat oven to 425°
Melt the butter as the oven preheats.
    Measure the flour into a large mixing bowl. Add baking powder, salt, and blueberries. Mix well. Put remaining ingredients into food processor or blender and blend until mixed. Then add to dry ingredients. Mix until just blended. Fill lined or lightly greased muffin tins two-thirds full. Bake for 25 minutes.
    Variations: Soy milk or water may be used in place of the milk. Honey or concentrated fruit juice may be used in place of the maple syrup. The egg can be eliminated or exchanged for egg replacer. Use one or a combination of other whole grain flours like barley, oat, buckwheat, millet, spelt, or kamut.

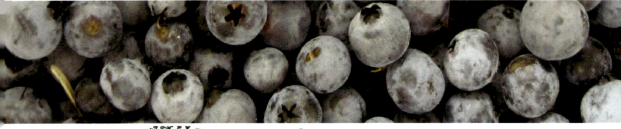

Spice of Life Specialty Foods PRESENTS

Zucchini Bread

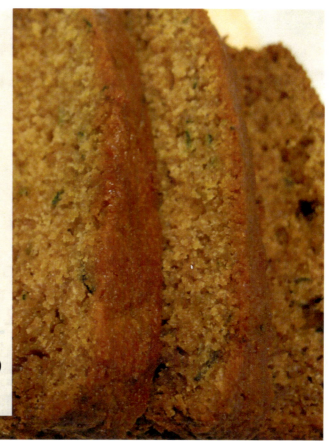

Makes 2 loaves

- ⅔ cup butter, softened (about 10 Tablespoons)
- ¾ cup honey
- ¾ cup maple syrup
- 4 eggs
- ⅓ cup milk, plain yogurt, or buttermilk
- 3 cups zucchini, shredded
- 3 cups unbleached flour
- 2 teaspoons baking soda
- 2 teaspoons sea salt
- 1 teaspoon baking powder
- 1 teaspoon ground cinnamon
- 1 teaspoon ground cloves
- 2 teaspoons vanilla
- ⅔ cup nuts, chopped (optional)
- ⅔ cup raisins (optional)

Preheat oven to 350°

Grease two loaf pans. In bowl of electric mixer, mix together the butter, honey, syrup, eggs, and milk. Add the zucchini. In another bowl, stir together the flour, soda, salt, baking powder, and spices. Blend the flour mixture into the wet ingredients. Add vanilla and beat until smooth. Stir in nuts and raisins if using. Divide into the two pans. Bake 1 hour and 10 minutes until a pick inserted into the center comes out clean. Cool slightly before removing from pans. Loosen sides of loaves from sides of pan before taking them out. Cool completely before slicing.

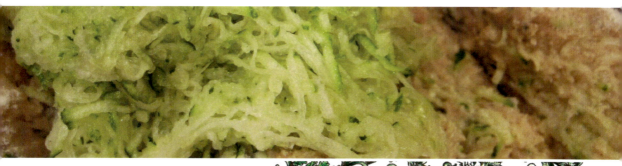

Finnish Cardamom Bread/Pulla/Nisu

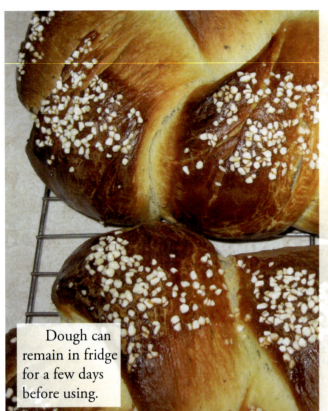

Dough can remain in fridge for a few days before using.

Makes 3 loaves

1⅓ cups milk
1⅓ cups hot water
1 cup organic sugar (or honey)
1 tablespoon active dry yeast
1 tablespoon sea salt
3 eggs
1 tablespoon cardamom, whole decorticated
1 stick butter, melted
8-9 cups unbleached flour

Topping:
1 egg, beaten
- pearl sugar to sprinkle on top (If this is not available at your grocery store, it may be found online, at World Market, or IKEA. Lars' Own is a brand imported from Sweden at IKEA.)

Into mixing bowl put milk, water, sugar, yeast, salt, and eggs. Grind cardamom in spice or coffee grinder and stir into other liquid mixture. Mix until eggs are beaten. Mix in the butter. Add flour a cup at a time and mix well by either using a mixer with a dough hook or by using your hand and a spoon. The dough should gather into a ball, but it can remain sticky. Cover dough with cloth, and put in a warm place to rise for one hour. After rising, pour out dough onto a lightly buttered counter or table top. With buttered hands, divide dough into three equal pieces (about 1½ pounds each). Form into loaves or braids (see below).

For braided pulla (nisu): Divide each piece into three parts. Form the 9 pieces into strands about 12 inches long and braid three strands together to end up with 3 loaves. Seal both ends and tuck under.

Place loaves on greased (or parchment papered) baking pan. Brush tops of loaves with beaten egg and sprinkle with pearl sugar. Let rise an additional 15-20 minutes in a warm place. Bake at 400° for 30 minutes.

Dough can also be used to make cinnamon rolls or small fruit-filled buns. See directions on following pages to complete either of these items. Each loaf size makes about 12 small rolls. Recipe is tweaked from *The Finnish Cookbook* by Beatrice Ojakangas.

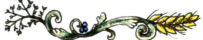

Spice of Life Specialty Foods **PRESENTS**

For Cinnamon Buns:

Makes 3 pie-sized sets of rolls

- 6 tablespoons butter
- ¼ cup maple syrup x3
- 2 tablespoons honey x3
- 2 tablespoons honey or maple sugar x3
- cinnamon to sprinkle
- 1 batch cardamom bread dough (page 58)

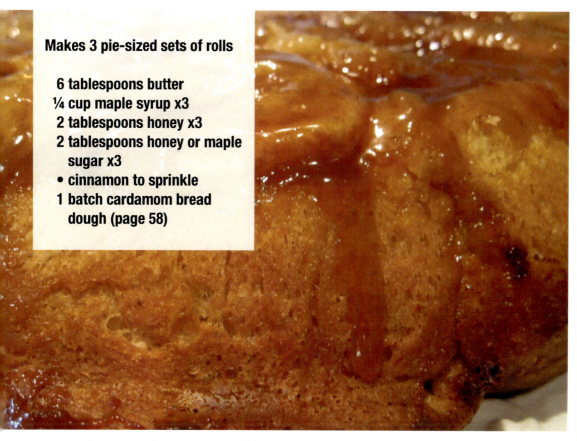

Preheat oven first to 200° and then to 375°.

Prepare three 9-inch pie or cake pans by putting 2 tablespoons butter in each pan. Pour over that, ¼ cup maple syrup and 2 tablespoons honey (for each pan). Put pans in warm 200° oven to melt butter. Divide dough into 3 parts. Working with one part of the dough at a time, roll or pat it out on a greased counter top into a rectangle 12x8 inches. Drizzle the surface with 2 tablespoons honey or maple sugar (for each pan). Sprinkle with cinnamon. Roll up and cut into one inch pieces. Place rolls in prepared pans. Increase oven temperature to 375°. Let rolls rise about 20 minutes. Bake at 375° for 25-30 minutes. When removing from oven, invert onto a large plate, and scrape out any leftover syrup, drizzling over the rolls.

For Fruit & Nut Filled Buns:

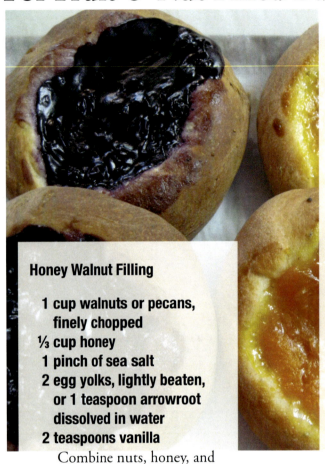

Fruit Filling

- 2 cups of your favorite fruit or berries like blueberries, raspberries, or rhubarb
- ½ cup water
- ¼ cup honey
- ¼ cup maple syrup
- 1 pinch of sea salt
- 2 tablespoons arrowroot starch
- 4 tablespoons cold water to dissolve arrowroot
- 2 tablespoons butter
- 2 teaspoons vanilla extract

In two quart sauce pan, bring berries, water, honey, maple syrup and salt to a boil. Watch carefully so it does not boil over. Frozen raspberries and strawberries need to be boiled just enough to thaw them. Blueberries need to cook about five minutes, and rhubarb about 10 minutes. Dissolve the arrowroot in four tablespoons of cold water, stirring until smooth. Add to the cooked fruit, and stir until thickened. Add butter and vanilla. Stir to mix. Allow to cool slightly before using to fill buns.

Honey Walnut Filling

- 1 cup walnuts or pecans, finely chopped
- ⅓ cup honey
- 1 pinch of sea salt
- 2 egg yolks, lightly beaten, or 1 teaspoon arrowroot dissolved in water
- 2 teaspoons vanilla

Combine nuts, honey, and salt in small saucepan. Bring to a boil. Thicken by gradually stirring in beaten egg yolks or arrowroot. Add vanilla.

Prepare buns using 1 batch of cardamom bread dough (page 58) for fruit filling and ⅓ batch for nut filling. Preheat oven to 375°

Divide each third of dough into 12 small balls and pat each one into a 4-inch round with the center flatter than the edge, similar to a pizza crust. The raised edge would be about ½" wide. Fill center depression with one heaping tablespoon of fruit or nut filling. Let prepared buns rise for 20 minutes. Bake at 375° for 25 minutes.

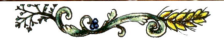

Spice of Life Specialty Foods PRESENTS

Cinnamon Rolls

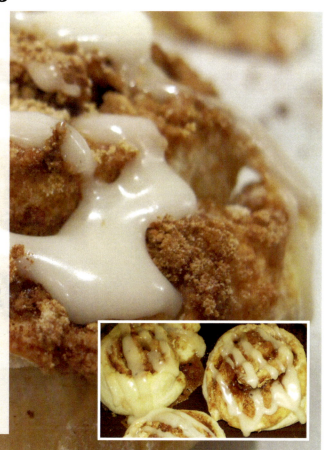

Makes 12 rolls

- ¼ stick butter, (2 tablespoons) softened to room temperature
- 1 cup unbleached flour
- 1 teaspoon baking powder
- ½ teaspoon sea salt
- 1 tablespoon yogurt
- ½ cup milk
- 1 tablespoon maple syrup
- ½ cup maple sugar (or organic sugar and more maple syrup)
- cinnamon to sprinkle

Icing:
- ½ cup powdered sugar
- ½ teaspoon vanilla
- 2 teaspoons milk

Preheat oven to 400°

Mix butter, flour, baking powder, and salt together. Add yogurt, milk, and maple syrup. Mix well. Roll dough out on floured counter to about a 12"x10" rectangle. Sprinkle maple sugar onto all of dough. (If using organic sugar, drizzle with maple syrup.) Sprinkle cinnamon on top of sugar. Roll dough up starting with 12" side. Cut into 12 slices. Turn slices on side and place on greased/parchment papered baking sheet. Bake for 13 minutes.

Mix icing ingredients together in fold-top sandwich bag. Using scissors, clip about ¼ inch off one bottom corner of the bag. Using this hole, squeeze out icing onto cinnamon rolls. Keep unused icing in the refrigerator.

Spaghetti

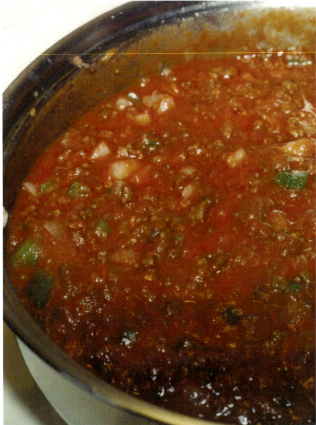

Homemade sauce has great flavor.

Serves 6-8

- 1 package spaghetti noodles (use amount to serve) try whole wheat for a change
- 1-2 pounds ground beef
- 1 medium onion
- 2-3 cloves garlic
- 1 green bell pepper or a mix of green, red, and yellow sweet pepper slices (optional)
- 2 tablespoons red wine (optional)
- 2 cans tomato sauce (look for sauce with peppers and onions)
- 1 can tomato paste
- 1 sprinkle of Trocomare® (seasoned salt)
- 1 tablespoon fresh parsley
- ½ teaspoon oregano
- ½ teaspoon basil
- 1 pinch thyme
- 1 pinch savory
- 1 pinch rosemary
- 1 pinch sage
- 2 tablespoons honey
- 1 pinch red pepper flakes
- 1 pinch fennel seed, ground

Brown ground beef in large frying pan over medium heat. Cut the onion and peppers into small pieces. Dice (or squeeze) the garlic. When meat is fully browned, add onion, peppers, and garlic, and fry until onions are translucent and soft. Add wine (optional). Add tomato sauce and paste and mix well. Add salt, parsley, oregano, basil, thyme, savory, rosemary, sage, honey, red pepper, and fennel. Stir. Cook for a few more minutes; then turn temperature down to low. Cook noodles following directions on package. Either serve separately or mix together.

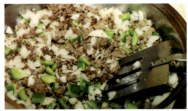
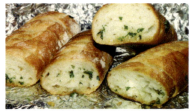
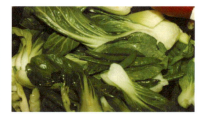

Spice of Life Specialty Foods PRESENTS

Turkey Rice Casserole

Serves 4-6

- 1 cup uncooked brown rice
- 1-2 cups cooked turkey, cubed
- 4 cups turkey broth
- 1 medium onion, chopped
- 1 clove garlic, minced
- 3 stalks celery, chopped
- 1 tablespoon parsley flakes
- 2 teaspoons paprika
- 2 teaspoons Trocomare® (seasoned salt)
- 1 small jar or can mushrooms (optional), sliced

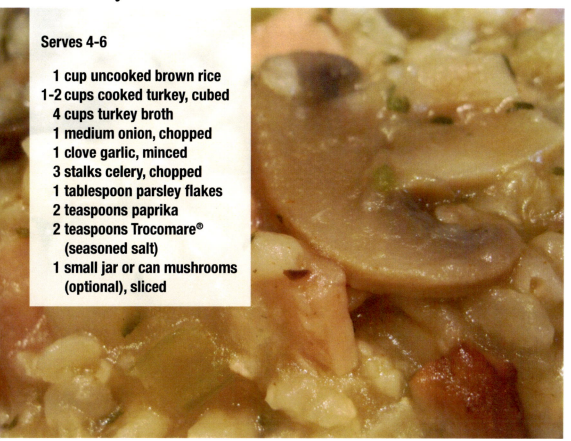

Preheat oven to 325°
Wash rice and put into 2-quart covered casserole or baking dish. Add remaining ingredients. Stir to mix. Cover and bake for 1½ to 2 hours. Stir after 1 hour. As baking time nears the end, add more water if needed.

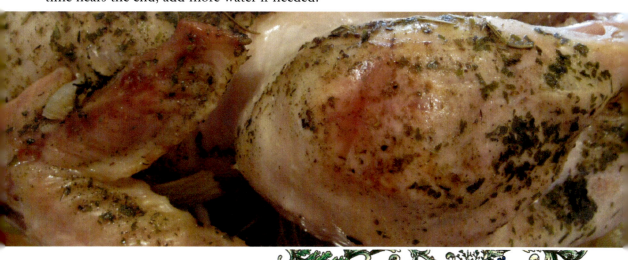

Marinade for Lamb Roast

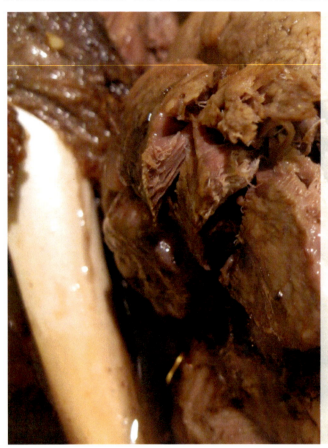

For 3-4 pound roast

- ⅔ cup berry or fruit juice OR ⅓ cup wine and ⅓ cup juice
- ⅓ cup tamari/soy sauce
- ¼ cup olive oil
- ½ teaspoon garlic powder
- ½ teaspoon onion powder
- 1 pinch red pepper flakes
- 1 bay leaf

Herbs to sprinkle before cooking
- basil
- oregano
- sage
- thyme
- rosemary
- savory
- marjoram

Mix ingredients together. Rub on roast. Allow to marinade refrigerated for at least 2 hours or up to 2 days. Before cooking, sprinkle with basil, oregano, sage, thyme, rosemary, savory, and marjoram. Cook roast according to instructions. Various cuts of lamb work well. Pictured here are lamb shanks. One cooking option is using a dutch oven and cooking between 275°-325° for 3-5 hours. Check to make sure liquid remains in pot. Check temperature to see when roast is done: 120°-185° varies from rare to well-done. If meat is falling off the bone, you have succeeded!

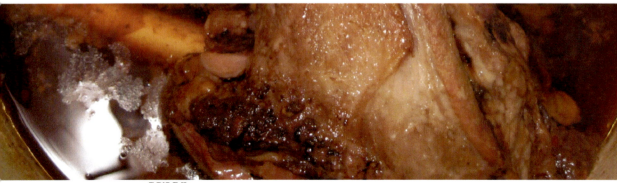

Spice of Life Specialty Foods PRESENTS

Marinade for Grilled Turkey

Makes 1 pint

- 1 medium onion
- 1 clove garlic
- ¼ cup tamari/soy sauce
- ¼ cup olive oil
- 1 tablespoon honey or maple syrup
- 1 teaspoon black pepper
- 1 teaspoon crushed red pepper
- ½ teaspoon cinnamon
- ½ teaspoon nutmeg
- 2 teaspoons dried sage
- 2 teaspoons dried thyme
- 1 teaspoon
- 2 teaspoons Trocomare® (seasoned salt) or sea salt
- 1 lemon, juice only

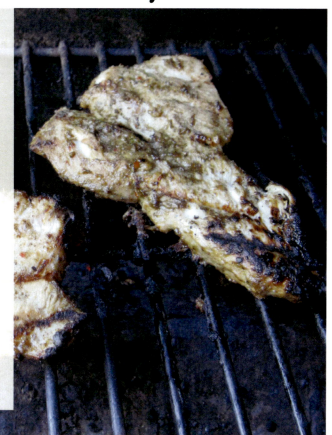

Blend all ingredients in blender. Coat about 3 pounds of turkey steaks or cubes, and allow to marinate several hours or overnight before grilling. Use 1½ pounds of turkey for half recipe of marinade or 3 pounds for full recipe.

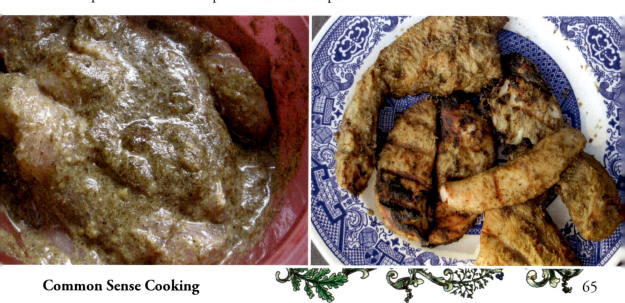

Common Sense Cooking

Grilled Whole Turkey

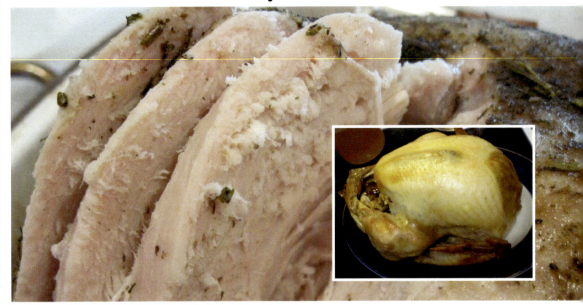

Cooking on the grill in the summer can be a wonderful opportunity to fix healthy foods for the family. A fresh turkey fixed on the grill with mesquite or hickory wood chips can easily stand up to ham flavor wise, but is without the excess salt.

Grilling a whole turkey requires a drip pan beneath it so that the meat is not directly over the coals dripping potentially harmful fat on them. The first step, though, is to heat the charcoal. For a 22-inch grill, you will need 50 briquettes. For an 18-inch diameter grill, use 32 briquettes. Heap them in the center of the lower shelf, and ignite them. For a smoked flavor, put 4 cups of mesquite, hickory or maple wood chips to soak in a bucket of water while the briquettes are heating. When the charcoal is coated with light gray ash, after about half an hour, divide the briquettes by moving half of them to each side of the lower rack. Position a flat drip pan or small roaster pan in the center between the coals below where the turkey will sit. Prepare the turkey for grilling by rinsing with cold water and patting dry. The turkey may be seasoned with salt and pepper, although it is not necessary. Tie the wings to the body with kitchen string or skewer pins. Also, make sure the legs are in the skin flap by the tail, or tie them together.

Put a large handful of the soaked wood chips over the charcoal on each side of the drip pan. Replace the top grill rack, and center the turkey over the drip pan. Cover and allow 11 minutes cooking time per pound. If the turkey is stuffed, allow 2 minutes extra per pound. After each half hour of cooking time, add 4 briquettes and another handful of wood chips to each side. (Add 3 briquettes for the 18-inch grill.) You can test the internal temperature of the meat with a meat thermometer, if desired. Mesquite and hickory wood chips add wonderful flavor when used as described above with any meat on the grill.

Spice of Life Specialty Foods **PRESENTS**

Basting Sauce or Marinade for Grilled Fish or Chicken

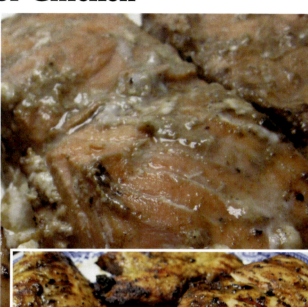

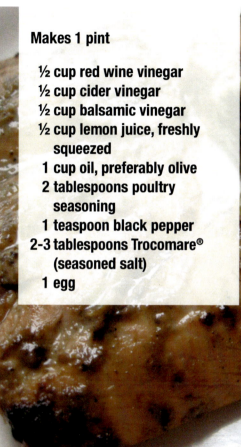

Makes 1 pint

- ½ cup red wine vinegar
- ½ cup cider vinegar
- ½ cup balsamic vinegar
- ½ cup lemon juice, freshly squeezed
- 1 cup oil, preferably olive
- 2 tablespoons poultry seasoning
- 1 teaspoon black pepper
- 2-3 tablespoons Trocomare® (seasoned salt)
- 1 egg

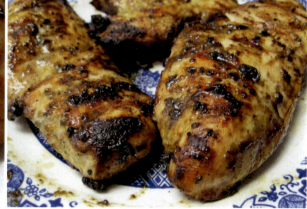

Put all ingredients into blender. Cover and blend on top speed until well mixed. This makes enough for several uses, so keep the extra in the refrigerator, and stir or shake well before using.

Several hours before grilling time, put thawed or fresh fish into a container big enough for the pieces to lie flat and soak up the marinade. Spoon some of the sauce over the fish. Turn the fish pieces over and spoon some more sauce so that they are coated in marinade. If possible, every half hour or so, turn the fish over and spoon the sauce from the bottom of the container onto the top of the fish. Grill fish for 4-5 minutes on each side. Drizzle with fresh lemon juice before serving.

The sauce may be used similarly for chicken—either breasts or cut up fryer pieces. Chicken pieces with skin on take longer to grill, so they can also be basted with the sauce while they are on the grill, every time you turn the pieces.

Grilled Chicken Marinades

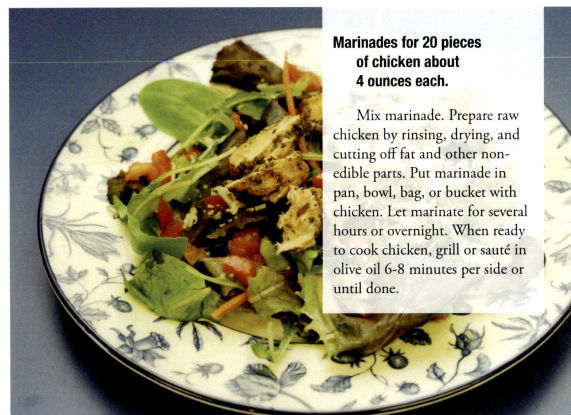

Marinades for 20 pieces of chicken about 4 ounces each.

Mix marinade. Prepare raw chicken by rinsing, drying, and cutting off fat and other non-edible parts. Put marinade in pan, bowl, bag, or bucket with chicken. Let marinate for several hours or overnight. When ready to cook chicken, grill or sauté in olive oil 6-8 minutes per side or until done.

Lemon Herb Marinade

- ¼ cup olive oil
- 2 lemons, juice only
- ½ cup balsamic vinegar
- 1 pinch red pepper flakes
- 1 tablespoon Trocomare® (seasoned salt)
- 6 tablespoons basil
- 6 tablespoons parsley
- 2 tablespoons oregano
- 1 tablespoon red wine vinegar

Teriyaki Marinade

- ¼ cup olive oil
- ⅓ cup tamari/soy sauce
- ⅓ cup red wine vinegar
- ⅓ cup black currant juice (or similar fruit or berry juice)
- 1 tablespoon balsamic vinegar
- 1 pinch red pepper flakes
- 1 tablespoon onion powder
- 3 large cloves garlic, crushed
- 1 large piece of ginger, peeled and grated

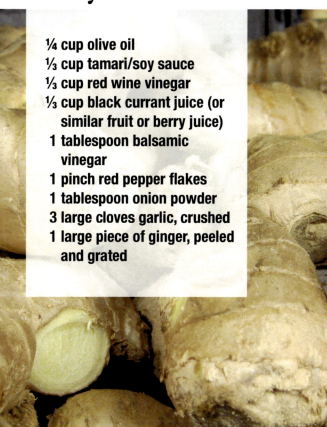

Spicy Marinade

- ¼ cup olive oil
- 1 tablespoon red wine vinegar
- 1 tablespoon balsamic vinegar
- ¼ cup tamari/soy sauce
- 1 tablespoon Trocomare® (seasoned salt)
- 1 tablespoon garlic granules
- 3 large cloves garlic, crushed
- 1 tablespoon onion powder or flakes
- 1 grapefruit, juice only (or 1 orange and 1 lemon or lime)
- 2 tablespoons maple syrup
- ¾ tablespoon allspice
- ¾ tablespoon thyme
- 1 teaspoon sage
- 1 teaspoon marjoram
- ¾ teaspoon cinnamon
- ¾ teaspoon nutmeg
- 1 pinch rosemary
- ½ teaspoon savory

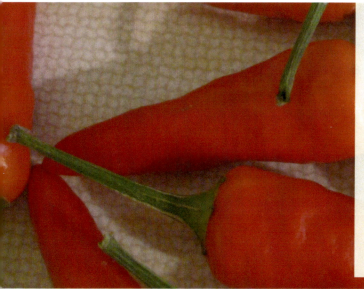

Common Sense Cooking

Baked Fish Fillets in Tomato Sauce

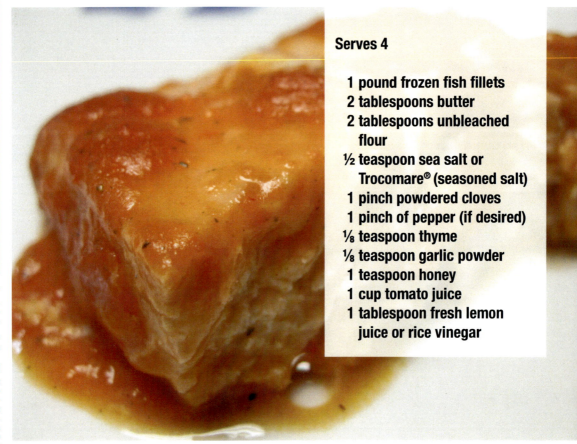

Serves 4

1 pound frozen fish fillets
2 tablespoons butter
2 tablespoons unbleached flour
½ teaspoon sea salt or Trocomare® (seasoned salt)
1 pinch powdered cloves
1 pinch of pepper (if desired)
⅛ teaspoon thyme
⅛ teaspoon garlic powder
1 teaspoon honey
1 cup tomato juice
1 tablespoon fresh lemon juice or rice vinegar

Preheat oven to 350°

In a small saucepan, melt the butter; blend in the flour, salt, cloves, pepper, thyme, garlic powder, and honey. Add tomato juice and cook, stirring constantly over medium high heat until mixture thickens. Add lemon juice and pour half of sauce into a shallow baking pan. Place slightly-thawed fish fillets over sauce. Top fish with remaining sauce. Bake in oven for 30-40 minutes, depending on the thickness of the fillets. After 15 minutes, the fish may be basted with the tomato sauce.

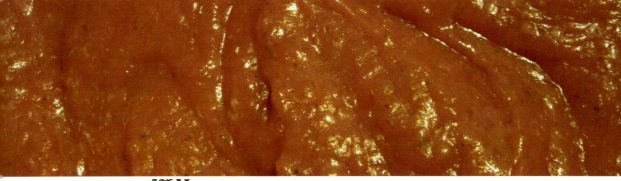

Potato Pancakes

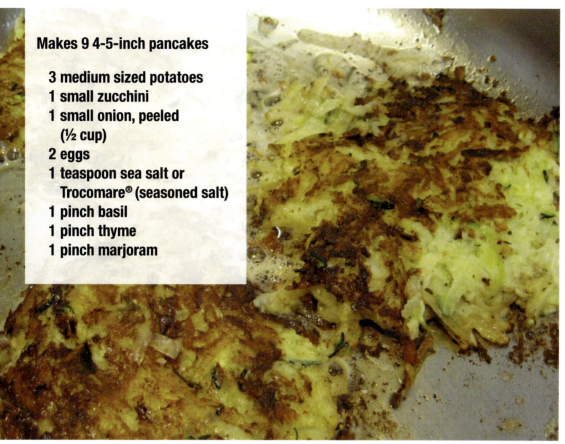

Makes 9 4-5-inch pancakes

- 3 medium sized potatoes
- 1 small zucchini
- 1 small onion, peeled (½ cup)
- 2 eggs
- 1 teaspoon sea salt or Trocomare® (seasoned salt)
- 1 pinch basil
- 1 pinch thyme
- 1 pinch marjoram

Scrub potatoes and peel if desired. Grate fine. Grate zucchini and onion. Mix grated vegetables together. Beat eggs and add to grated vegetables along with salt and herbs. Cook on a heavy greased skillet at medium heat/300° until brown on both sides. Put into 200° oven to stay warm and cook further until serving time.

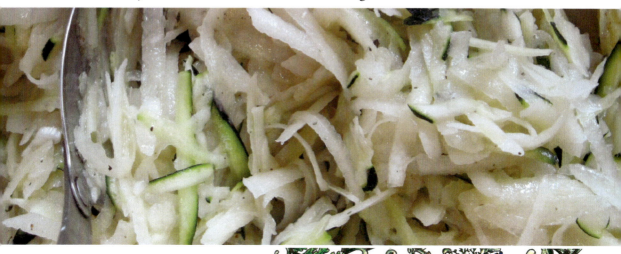

Seafood Lasagna

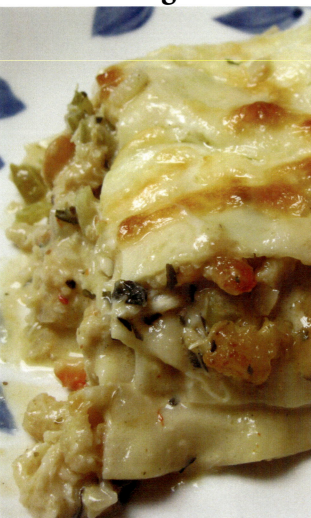

Fits 9x13 pan

- 3 cups onion, chopped
- 2 cups celery, chopped
- 2 cloves garlic, minced
- 2 tablespoons butter or olive oil
- ½ pound fresh mushrooms, cleaned and sliced, OR
- 4 ounces canned mushrooms
- 7 9-inch lasagna noodles
- 1 tablespoon olive oil
- 3 tablespoons arrow root or tapioca starch
- 2 cups milk or soy milk
- 2 teaspoons basil
- 2 teaspoons parsley
- ½ teaspoon savory
- ½ teaspoon marjoram
- ½ teaspoon paprika
- 1 tablespoon tamari/soy sauce
- 2 teaspoons Trocomare® (seasoned salt)
- 1 dash of crushed red pepper
- 2 4-ounce cans of shrimp
- 1 6-ounce can of crab
- ½ cup cream cheese or soymage sour cream
- 8 ounces cheddar cheese (or soy cheese), grated

Saute the onion, celery and garlic in the butter or oil about 5 minutes. Add mushrooms and cook five minutes more. Cook lasagna noodles in a large kettle in 3 quarts of water with 1 tablespoon oil for 12 minutes. Drain noodles and cool. Dissolve starch in milk. Add milk mixture to onion-mushroom mixture and stir over medium heat until thickened. Season with herbs, soy sauce, Trocomare®, and pepper. Drain and rinse the shrimp and crab meat; add it to the mushroom sauce. Stir in cream cheese. In a 9x13 cake or lasagna pan, spread a thin layer of the shrimp-mushroom sauce. Top with a layer of noodles. Alternate layers of sauce and noodles until they are all used up. Top with grated cheese. Bake at 350° for 45 minutes. Allow to stand 15 minutes before serving.

Lasagna

Fits 10x14 pan

- 1 pound mild Italian sausage
- 2 pounds lean ground beef
- 1 tablespoon olive oil
- 1 large onion, chopped
- 2 large cloves garlic, minced
- 3 16-ounce cans or jars tomato sauce
- 1 tablespoon fennel seed, partly ground
- 2 teaspoons chili powder
- 2 teaspoons Trocomare® (seasoned salt)
- 2 tablespoons parsley
- 1 tablespoon basil
- 1 tablespoon maple syrup or honey
- 8 ounces lasagna noodles (10 noodles)
- 4 quarts boiling water
- 1 tablespoon olive oil
- 2 teaspoons sea salt
- 2 pounds ricotta cheese
- 3 eggs
- 2 tablespoons parsley flakes
- ½ teaspoon Trocomare®
- ¼ teaspoon black pepper
- ¾ pound mozzarella cheese, sliced or grated
- ½ cup grated Romano or Parmesan cheese

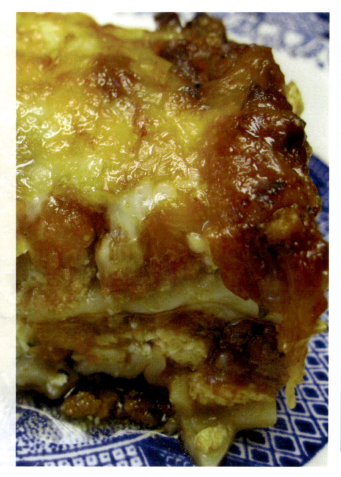

Preheat oven to 350°

Brown the meat and drain off excess fat. Stir in olive oil, onion, and garlic and cook until soft. Then add tomato sauce and seasonings: fennel, chili powder, Trocomare®, parsley, basil, and maple syrup. Simmer one hour.

Meanwhile, cook noodles in boiling water with oil and salt for about 10-12 minutes. Rinse and drain. Mix ricotta, eggs, parsley, Trocomare®, and pepper.

In large lasagna pan put thin layer of sauce, then half of the noodles. Put a layer of ricotta and a layer of meat sauce. Cover with mozzarella. Put rest of noodles, ricotta, meat sauce and mozzarella. Sprinkle top with Romano. Bake for 45 minutes. Let stand 15 minutes before serving.

Fried Fish

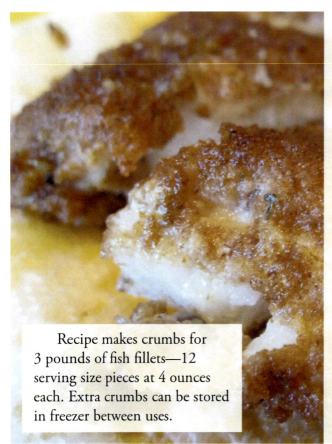

- 1½ cups cracker crumbs
- 1 tablespoon Trocomare® (seasoned salt)
- 1 tablespoon paprika
- 1 tablespoon dried parsley
- 1 tablespoon garlic powder or granules
- 1 tablespoon onion powder
- 2 teaspoons basil
- 2 teaspoons oregano
- 2 teaspoons ground thyme
- 2 teaspoons marjoram
- 1 teaspoon ground rosemary
- 1 teaspoon ground sage
- 1 teaspoon ground savory

- 1 egg per 2 fillets
- fish fillets of your choice (if frozen, thaw for 1-2 hours)
- oil or butter for cooking
- fresh lemon for serving

Recipe makes crumbs for 3 pounds of fish fillets—12 serving size pieces at 4 ounces each. Extra crumbs can be stored in freezer between uses.

MAIN DISHES

In blender make crumbs from your choice of crackers and one slice of bread toasted and dried crisp. For example, use nut thins, hardtack, Finn Crisp, and/or rice cakes. Blend one type of broken crackers at a time until they are fine crumbs. Pour out into a bowl until you have the full amount. Then mix in seasonings. Cut fish fillets into serving size pieces. In shallow bowl, whisk 1 egg until thoroughly blended. In another shallow bowl, put ⅔ cup of prepared crumbs (add more as needed). Dip fish pieces one at a time in beaten egg turning and poking it with a fork to absorb egg. Then dip the fish pieces in the crumbs and spoon some crumbs over the top. Fry at medium high heat in coconut oil, olive oil, butter, or a combination of favorite oils until browned on outside and fish flakes when cut. Squeeze fresh lemon and serve. Or serve with fresh lemon wedges.

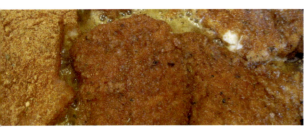
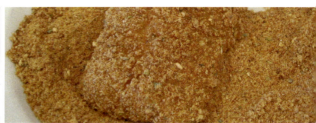

Spice of Life Specialty Foods PRESENTS

Lamb or Beef Meatballs

Serves 6

1 egg
1 slice onion
1 small garlic clove
2 tablespoons dijon mustard
½ teaspoon ground coriander
½ teaspoon ground allspice
¼ cup half and half
1 slice bread
1½ pound lean ground meat
• olive oil

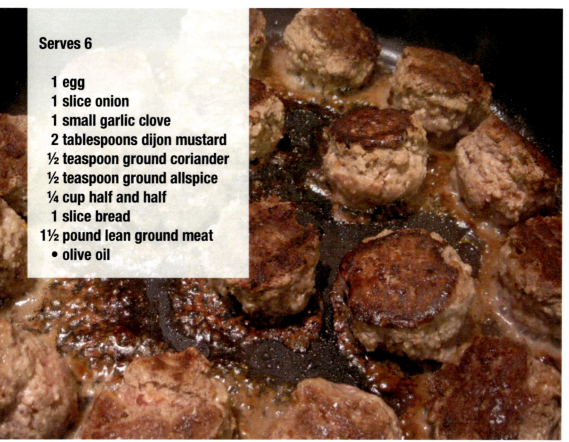

Place egg, onion, garlic, mustard, coriander, allspice, cream, and bread into a blender. Cover and blend until smooth. Pour into a mixing bowl along with the ground meat. Mix well. Shape into balls, and cook in a hot skillet using olive oil as needed.

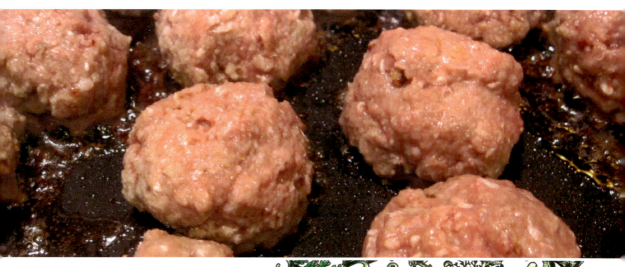

Turkey Meatballs

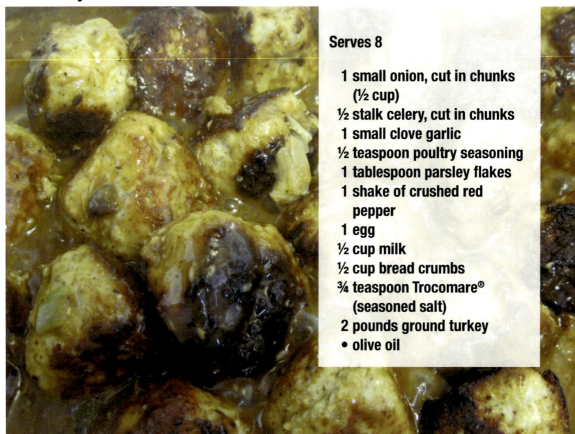

Serves 8

- 1 small onion, cut in chunks (½ cup)
- ½ stalk celery, cut in chunks
- 1 small clove garlic
- ½ teaspoon poultry seasoning
- 1 tablespoon parsley flakes
- 1 shake of crushed red pepper
- 1 egg
- ½ cup milk
- ½ cup bread crumbs
- ¾ teaspoon Trocomare® (seasoned salt)
- 2 pounds ground turkey
- olive oil

In blender, combine onion, celery, garlic, poultry seasoning, parsley, red pepper, egg, milk, bread crumbs, and Trocomare®. Cover and blend until smooth. Pour into a mixing bowl along with the ground turkey. Mix well. Shape into balls, and brown in a hot skillet using olive oil as needed. Remove meatballs from pan onto a platter when brown. When all meatballs are browned, make a mushroom gravy either from scratch (see page 77) or from a dry mix without MSG. Then return the meatballs to the gravy and simmer ten minutes. Serve with rice, potatoes, or pasta.

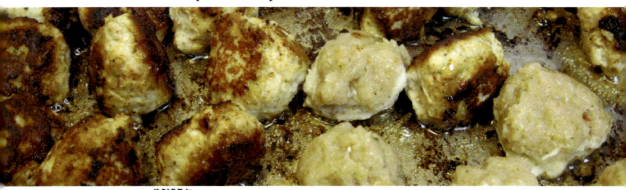

Spice of Life Specialty Foods PRESENTS

Mushroom Sauce

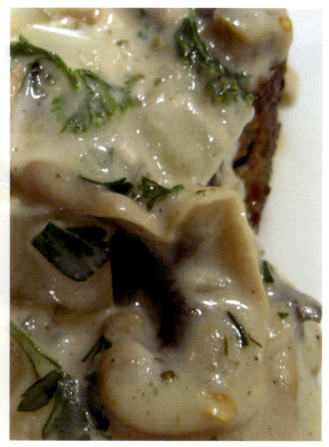

Makes 1 pint

- 1 medium onion, chopped fine
- 2 cloves garlic, minced
- 1 8-ounce package mushrooms, sliced or chopped
- 4 tablespoons butter or olive oil
- 2 cups milk or half and half
- 2 tablespoons arrowroot or kuzu starch
- 1 dash crushed red pepper
- 1 tablespoon tamari/soy sauce
- ½ teaspoon thyme
- ½ teaspoon marjoram
- ½ teaspoon savory
- ½ teaspoon paprika
- 2 teaspoons parsley flakes
- 1 teaspoon Trocomare® (seasoned salt)

Saute onions, garlic, and mushrooms in butter or oil until tender. Dissolve arrowroot starch in milk, add to vegetables and heat slowly to boiling, stirring occasionally until thick. Add seasonings. Taste for salt, adding more if desired. May substitute soy, rice, or almond milk.

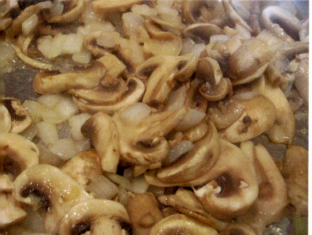
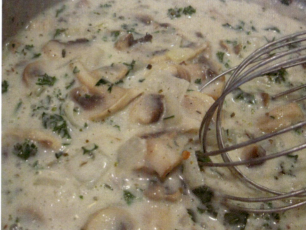

Finnish Karelian Pastries/Karjalan Piirakkas

Kar·ja·lan Pii·rak·ka: Kuhr´-yuh-lahn Pee´-ruh-kuh
(p is actually mix between p and b, and roll the r)

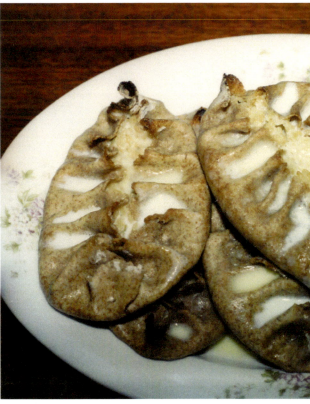

Makes 12

2 cups water
1 teaspoon sea salt
1½ cups brown rice
2 cups milk
2 tablespoons butter

Crust:
2 tablespoons butter
1 cup very hot water
1 teaspoon sea salt
1 cup unbleached flour
2 cups rye flour

Basting Sauce:
½ cup hot milk
2 tablespoons butter

Preheat oven to 450°
In a 3 quart kettle (or larger), bring the water to a boil. Add salt and rice. Reduce heat, cover, and cook half an hour.

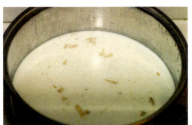

Add the milk one cup at a time and cook covered until the rice is done and the milk is absorbed. This can take from 45 minutes to more than 1½ hour. Stir in the butter.

While the rice is cooking, make the crust. In a large mixing bowl, melt the butter in very hot water. Add salt. Add the unbleached flour and mix well. Add one cup of rye flour and mix in. The second cup of rye flour may need to be mixed in by hand and kneaded as

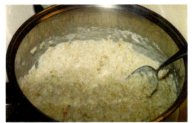
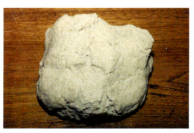

Spice of Life Specialty Foods PRESENTS

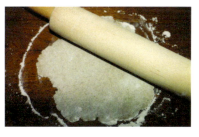

for bread dough at the end. The dough should be soft and smooth.

On a floured rolling surface, cut the dough into 12 equal sized portions. Taking one at a time, pat it into a small round. Then rolling from the center out to the edges in each direction, roll to about a 7-inch circle, keeping it as round as possible.

Put rolled dough circles onto cooking parchment or greased cookie sheets. When the filling is cooked, put 3 tablespoons filling on each circle of dough. Spread filling out to about an inch from the edge. Bring up two opposite sides of the dough, one with each hand, and pinch together between the thumb and forefinger a small crimp or pleat in the dough the same on both sides. Lay the edges of the dough about an inch apart on the rice filling so that there will be an inch wide strip of rice filling exposed in the middle. Work from the first crimp and make additional crimps in the edges of the dough on both sides up to the top of the round and again starting

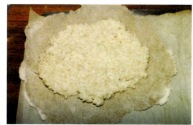

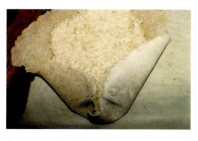

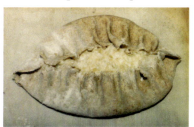

from the first crimp, work down to the bottom so you end up with an oval-shaped pastry, the crimps having taken up the slack of the circle. You can fit four of them on a cookie sheet at a time. When they are filled and crimped, bake for 15 minutes while you make the next panful. When the pastries are baked, dip them for a few seconds into a pan of basting sauce made from hot milk in which butter is melted. Remove from basting sauce onto a serving platter. Serve hot or cold with mashed hardboiled eggs, cheese, cold cuts, or just butter.

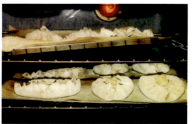

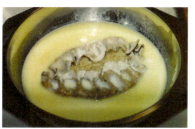

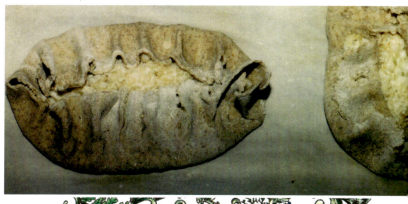

Common Sense Cooking

Pasty

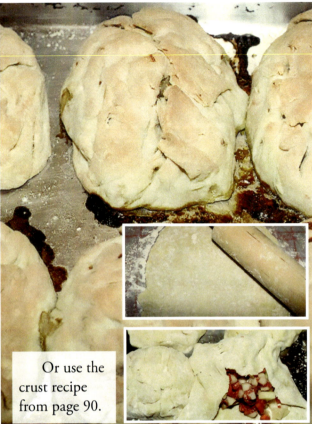

Makes 6 pasties

- 6 potatoes (medium-4 ½"), 6 cups chopped ½" cubes
- 3 carrots, ¾ cup chopped fine
- 1 stalk celery, ⅔ cup chopped fine
- 1 onion, 1 cup chopped fine
- 1 large clove garlic, minced (optional)
- 1½ pounds ground beef (or chopped steak)
- 1½ tablespoon Trocomare® (seasoned salt)
- ½ teaspoon black pepper

Crust:
- 3 sticks butter
- 6 cups unbleached flour
- 1 tablespoon Trocomare® (seasoned salt)
- 2 eggs
- 2 tablespoons vinegar
- 1 cup water

Or use the crust recipe from page 90.

Mix butter, flour and 1 tablespoon Trocomare® (or seasoned salt) with a pastry blender. Whisk together egg, vinegar, and water. Add to flour mixture and mix into ball. Let stand while cutting vegetables. Mix vegetables, optional garlic, beef, 1½ tablespoons Trocomare®, and pepper in a large bowl. Use clean hands and mix the beef in well.

Preheat oven to 375°

Divide dough into 6 equal pieces. Find a clean, floured area, and using a floured rolling pin, roll carefully into thin 10-12" circles. Divide vegetable mix and put a serving onto each piece of dough. (About 1½ cups.) Pull up and seal dough edges. Or place vegetable mix on one side of dough circle and pull other half of dough circle over top and seal the two pieces where they come together. Place on baking pan. Pasties will leak; use a baking sheet with a lip so liquid doesn't drip into oven. Bake for one hour.

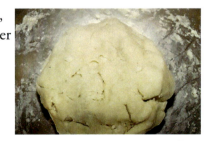

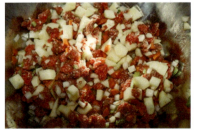

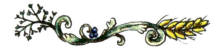

Spice of Life Specialty Foods PRESENTS

Pizza from Scratch

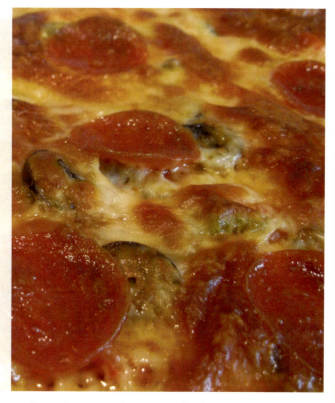

Makes 2 pizzas

- 1 package active dry yeast
- 1 tablespoon honey
- 1 teaspoon sea salt
- 2 cups warm water
- 2 cups whole grain flour
- 3 cups unbleached flour
- 1 pint tomato sauce
- 1 can tomato paste
- 1 teaspoon oregano
- 1 tablespoon parsley
- 1 teaspoon marjoram
- 1 teaspoon basil
- ½ teaspoon savory
- 1 teaspoon fennel seed, ground

Toppings:

- 1 pound shredded mozzarella cheese
- sweet onion, sliced
- green pepper, thinly sliced
- mushroom, sliced
- black olives, sliced
- 1 pound turkey Italian sausage, sliced and browned (optional)

Dissolve yeast, honey, and salt in warm water in a medium size mixing bowl. Add whole grain flour and mix well. Add unbleached flour a cup at a time and stir until a soft dough forms. Grease the top of the dough and allow to rise about an hour. Punch down dough, and divide into two equal parts. Grease two pizza pans or cookie sheets. With greased hands, pat the dough out evenly onto the pans forming a thicker rim around the edges. Allow to rise ten minutes. Bake at 425° for ten minutes. If desired, after the crust bakes, lift it off the pan and turn it over. The sauce will soak into the crust instead of rolling off.

Combine the tomato sauce and paste. Stir in the herbs. Divide the sauce between the two pizzas. Top with desired vegetables and then the cheese. Bake for ten to fifteen minutes—until cheese is melted and pizza is hot through.

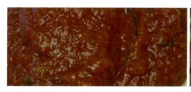
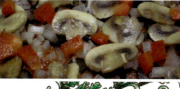
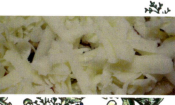

Rhubarb Custard Pie

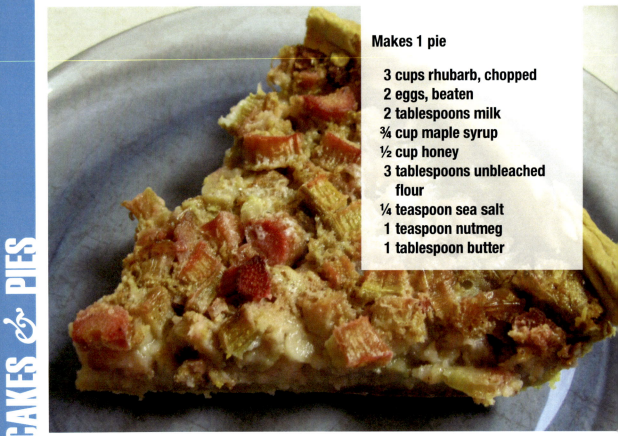

Makes 1 pie

3 cups rhubarb, chopped
2 eggs, beaten
2 tablespoons milk
¾ cup maple syrup
½ cup honey
3 tablespoons unbleached flour
¼ teaspoon sea salt
1 teaspoon nutmeg
1 tablespoon butter

Preheat oven to 375°
   Spread rhubarb into unbaked pie crust (page 90). Put eggs, milk, maple syrup, honey, flour, sea salt, and nutmeg in blender. Blend until well mixed. Pour over rhubarb. Dot with butter. Bake for 15 minutes. Reduce heat to 350° and bake for 35-40 minutes.
   Recipe is originally from Sarah Katherine Maki.

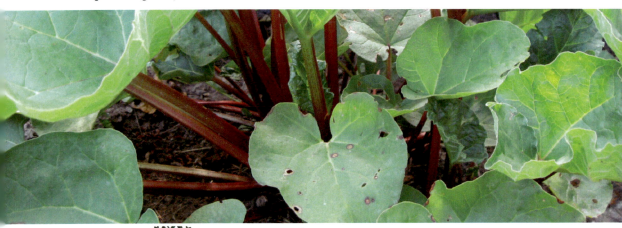

Spice of Life Specialty Foods PRESENTS

Baked Cheesecake

Fits in a 9x9 pan

Crust:
½ package Leibniz Butter Biscuits (7-ounce full package), crushed in blender, food processor, or with rolling pin,
OR other butter cookies
½ stick butter, melted

Filling:
19 ounces cream cheese, softened to room temperature
1 cup organic sugar
½ lemon, juice only
1 teaspoon vanilla
3 eggs

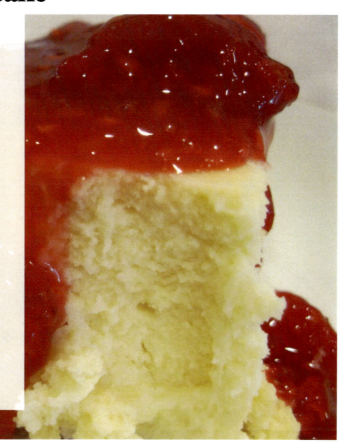

Preheat oven to 300°

Mix crushed cookies with butter. Press into bottom of 9x9 glass pan. Put in freezer until filling is ready. In mixer, beat cream cheese and sugar together until smooth. Add lemon and vanilla. Add eggs one at a time beating on low until just mixed in. Pour into crust. Bake for one hour only. Cut into nine pieces.

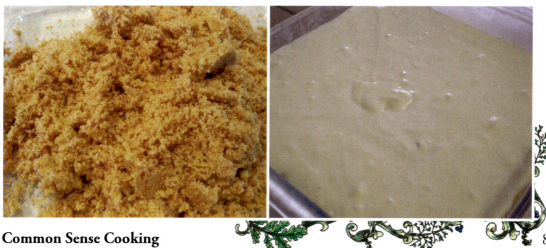

Common Sense Cooking

No-Bake Strawberry Cheesecake

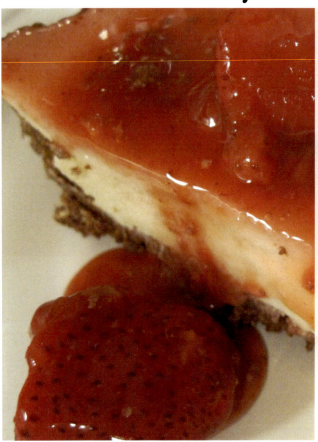

Makes 1 cake

18-ounce package graham crackers
1 stick butter, softened (½ cup: 8 tablespoons)
¼ cup cold milk
2 envelopes unflavored gelatin
¼ cup hot milk
½ cup honey or maple syrup
2 eggs (optional)
1 teaspoon vanilla
16 ounces plain yogurt
1 quart fresh strawberries
½ cup honey or maple syrup
1 teaspoon unflavored gelatin
1 tablespoon arrowroot starch
1 teaspoon butter
1 teaspoon vanilla

In a food processor, blend the graham crackers into crumbs. Mix with soft butter. Press into a 9-inch cake pan. Chill crust while preparing the cheesecake. Into the blender or food processor, put cold milk. Sprinkle in the gelatin. Let sit for 5 minutes. Then cover and blend. Add hot milk and blend again. Add sweetener, eggs and vanilla. Blend awhile; then scrape down any gelatin that wants to stick to the sides of the blender. Blend in the yogurt until smooth. Pour on top of chilled crust. Cover with a plastic wrap and chill until firm. Top with glazed strawberry topping and allow to chill before serving.

For strawberry glaze: Mash 1 cup of fresh berries. Put into small saucepan with honey or maple syrup and gelatin. Heat to boiling. Stir to dissolve gelatin. Dissolve 1 tablespoon arrowroot starch in cold water. Add to hot strawberry mixture. Cook while stirring until thickened. Stir in butter and vanilla. Arrange the remaining 3 cups of strawberries, whole or sliced, over top of firm cheesecake. Pour glaze over and chill before serving. Or mix remaining strawberries into cooked glaze and serve cheesecake with scoops of berry topping over each serving.

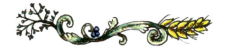

Spice of Life Specialty Foods PRESENTS

Raspberry-Filled Cake

Makes 16 servings

Cake:
- 1 cup unbleached flour, sifted
- 2 tablespoons cornstarch
- 1 teaspoon baking powder
- ¼ teaspoon sea salt
- 4 eggs
- 1 cup organic sugar

Raspberry Sauce:
- 4 cups frozen raspberries
- ¾ cup organic sugar
- 3 tablespoons cornstarch melted in water (about 2-3 tablespoons water)
- 1 teaspoon butter
- 1 teaspoon vanilla

Whipped Cream:
- 2 cups whipping cream
- ¼ cup maple sugar
- ¼ teaspoon vanilla

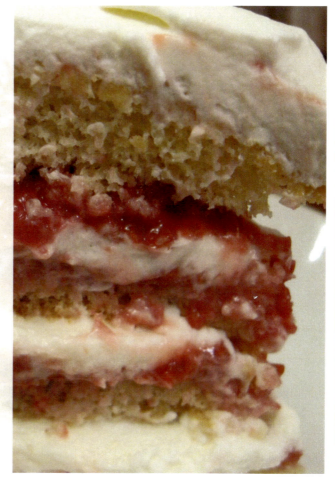

Preheat oven to 350°

Mix flour, 2 tablespoons cornstarch, baking powder, and salt in bowl. Set aside. In mixer, beat eggs until fluffy. Add 1 cup sugar and beat until thick—at least 5 minutes. Carefully fold the dry ingredients into the egg and sugar mixture making sure it is fully mixed. Pour the batter into a buttered 9x13 pan. Bake for 25 minutes.

Cook 2 cups raspberries with ¾ cup sugar and cornstarch. Continue stirring until thick. Melt butter in mixture and add 1 teaspoon vanilla. Then add the other 2 cups of frozen raspberries to cool it down.

Whip cream until thick. Beat in maple sugar and ¼ teaspoon vanilla. Cut cake horizontally in two layers. On top of bottom layer, spread half of the raspberry sauce and then about half of the whipped cream. Put the top layer of cake on upside down and spread on the rest of the raspberry sauce and whipped cream.
Cut into 16 servings.

Raspberry Cream Pie

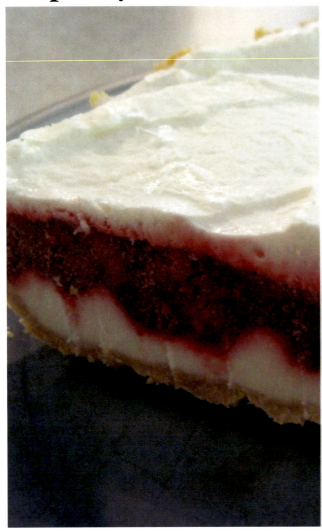

Makes 1 pie

Crust (1st Layer):
½ package Leibniz Butter Biscuits (7 oz full pkg), broken in blender or crushed with rolling pin
OR other butter cookies
½ stick butter, melted

Cream Cheese (2nd Layer):
8 ounces cream cheese, softened to room temperature
3 tablespoons maple syrup
1 teaspoon vanilla
1 tablespoon cream

Raspberry Sauce (3rd Layer):
3 cups frozen raspberries
¾ cup organic sugar
3 tablespoons cornstarch melted in water (about 3 tablespoons water)
1 tablespoon butter
1 teaspoon vanilla

Topping (4th Layer):
½ cup whipping cream
2 tablespoons maple sugar

Mix cookie crumbs and melted butter. Pat into bottom of 9" round or square pan. Mix cream cheese, maple syrup, vanilla, and cream in a mixer or food processor until smooth. Spread this cream cheese mixture over cookie crumbs making sure the crumbs are completely covered.

Mix 2 cups raspberries, sugar and cornstarch in saucepan. Cook while stirring until sauce changes from bright and milky to dark, glossy, and thick. Add butter and vanilla. Add the other cup of frozen raspberries to cool sauce. Pour over cream cheese as much or as little as desired.

Whip cream in mixer until thick. Whip in maple sugar. Put on top of raspberry sauce. Pie can be refrigerated until served. Also works great as individual servings in small tart pans.

Raspberry Sauce

Makes 5 cups

- 8 cups frozen raspberries
- 1½ cups organic sugar
- 4 tablespoons cornstarch
- ½ cup cold water
- 2 tablespoons butter
- ½ teaspoon vanilla

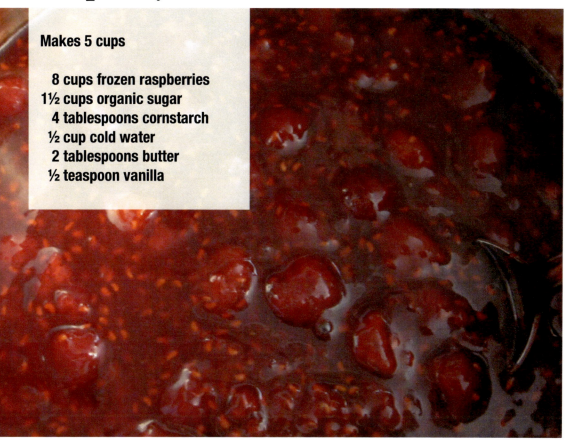

Pour 4 cups frozen raspberries into large pot. Add sugar. Heat slowly over medium-low heat until thawed. Dissolve cornstarch in cold water. Add to raspberries. Cook while stirring so sauce does not burn. Cook until starch is cooked and berries are thickened. If you wish, you can increase the heat, but be careful sauce does not burn. Add butter and vanilla. Stir in. Add rest of frozen berries and stir in. Use for pancakes, waffles or toast.

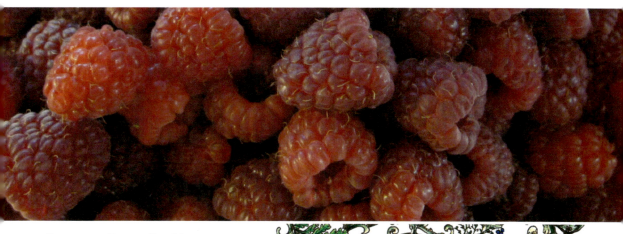

Carrot Cake

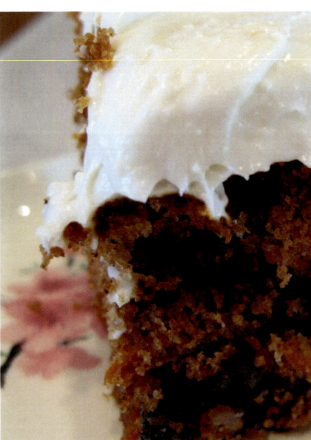

Makes 1 13x9 cake

- 1 cup whole wheat pastry flour
- 1 cup unbleached flour
- 2 teaspoons baking soda
- 2 teaspoons cinnamon
- ½ teaspoon sea salt
- ½ cup butter, soft
- ½ cup honey
- ½ cup maple syrup
- 2 eggs
- 1½ cups carrots, shredded
- ½ cup nuts

Frosting (Optional)
- 8 ounces cream cheese
- 1 tablespoon honey
- 1 tablespoon maple syrup
- 2 teaspoons vanilla

Preheat oven to 350°

Combine flour, baking soda, cinnamon, and salt in a bowl. Cream butter, honey, and maple syrup in a separate bowl, beating well. Add eggs and carrots. Beat again. Then fold in dry ingredients and nuts. Mix a minute or two until batter is velvety. Bake in a greased 13x9 pan for 30-35 minutes. Serve with or without cream cheese frosting made by mixing the cream cheese, honey, syrup, and vanilla. Cream cheese mixes best when room temperature and using a mixer or food processor.

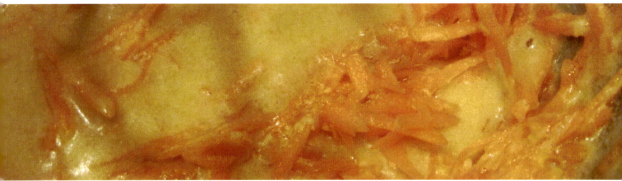

Our Favorite Fruit Cake

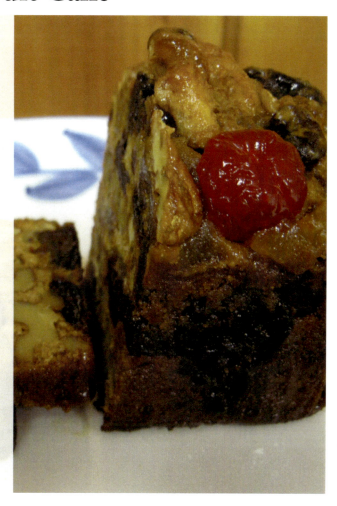

Makes 2 loaves

- 1½ cups unbleached flour
- 1½ cups organic sugar
- 1 teaspoon baking powder
- 1 teaspoon sea salt
- 1 8-ounce package raisins or dried cranberries
- 1 8-ounce package pitted dates, chopped
- 1 8-ounce package candied pineapple, cut up
- 4 8-ounce jars red cherries, drained (or 3 red and 1 green)
- 5½ cups walnut and pecans, halves and pieces (do not cut up)
- 6 eggs
- 1 ounce vanilla extract
- 1 ounce rum extract

Glaze:
- maple syrup
- rum (or rum extract)

Preheat oven to 300°

In a large mixing bowl, put flour, sugar, baking powder, salt, raisins, dates, pineapple, cherries, and nuts, and toss to mix. Put eggs and extracts into blender and mix well. Add egg mixture to dry mixture and stir until well mixed. Line two loaf pans with baking parchment. Pack the mixture tightly into the two pans. Bake one hour and 45 minutes. Cool 15 minutes and remove from pans. When cooled, remove parchment paper and glaze with maple syrup flavored with rum. After glazing, wrap in plastic wrap and turn cakes as they absorb the glaze.

For Christmas, we double the recipe and bake in small pans to give for gifts. The double recipe makes 11 of the 5 ½ x 2 ½. Or you can use some smaller ones as well. The large Texas-sized muffin papers make good liners for the small pans. The smaller pans bake for 1 hour and 10 minutes.

Common Sense Cooking

Pie Crust / Gluten-free Pie Crust

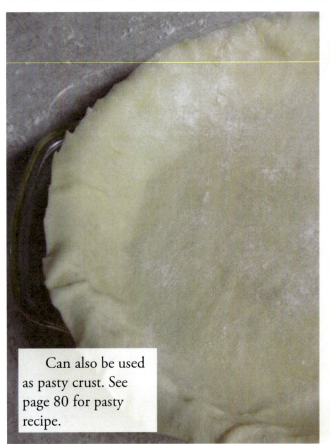

Can also be used as pasty crust. See page 80 for pasty recipe.

Makes four pie crusts.

Recipe is for prune tarts from the *Finnish Cookbook*.

¾ cup whipping cream
1 pinch of sea salt
1½ cup unbleached flour
½ teaspoon baking powder
½ cup butter, softened
 (1 stick: 8 tablespoons)

Makes two gluten-free crusts.

⅜ cup whipping cream
1 pinch of sea salt
¼ cup millet flour
¼ cup quinoa flour
¼ cup brown rice flour
½ teaspoon baking powder
2 tablespoons xanthan gum
2 teaspoons guar gum
¼ cup butter, softened
 (½ stick: 4 tablespoons)

Whip the cream until stiff. Sift together flour (flours, xanthan gum, and guar gum for gluten-free), salt, and baking powder. Mix in with cream until thoroughly blended. Stir in butter until blended. You can use a mixer with a dough hook. Chill for several hours (gluten-free let it rest for about 20 minutes) before rolling crusts out. You can make a half recipe for only two pies, but the dough will keep for a while in the fridge and longer in the freezer. When ready to make pie, roll out dough on floured surface, using floured rolling pin. Roll from center to edges, flipping and turning as you go adding more flour if necessary so crust doesn't stick to surface. For the gluten-free crust, roll and pat dough between plastic wrap layers. For a 9" pie pan, roll out a 12" circle.

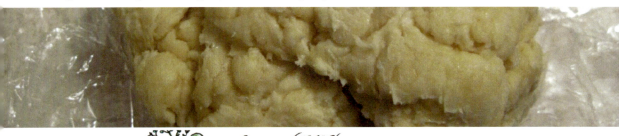

Pumpkin Pie

Makes one pie

- 2 cups squash or pumpkin, cooked
- ⅓ cup honey
- ⅓ cup maple syrup
- 3 eggs
- ¾ cup milk, cream, or half and half—any combination
- 1½ teaspoons cinnamon
- ½ teaspoon sea salt
- ½ teaspoon ginger
- ½ teaspoon nutmeg
- ½ teaspoon cloves

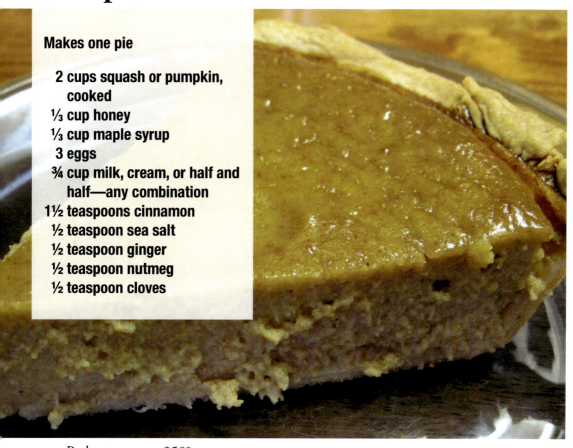

Preheat oven to 350°

Put all ingredients in the blender and blend until smooth. Then pour into a crust (page 90) and bake for 55-60 minutes.

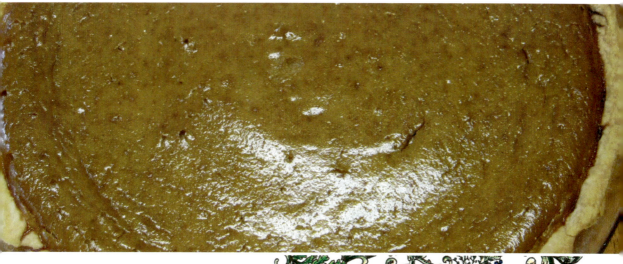

Bavarian Cream Pie

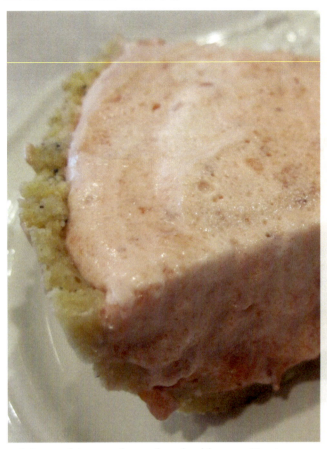

Makes 1 pie

Crust:
 ½ stick butter, melted
 ½ package Leibniz Butter Biscuits (7 oz full pkg), broken in blender or crushed with rolling pin
OR other butter cookies

Filling:
 1 quart strawberries or raspberries
 1 cup organic sugar
 2 teaspoons gelatin
 2 tablespoons water
 3 tablespoons water, boiling
 1 tablespoon lemon juice (optional)
 1 cup whipping cream
 1 tablespoon maple syrup
 1 teaspoon vanilla

Mix cookie crumbs and melted butter. Pat into bottom of 9" round or square pan.

If frozen, thaw berries. Mash berries in sugar and let stand 30 minutes. Dissolve gelatin in water. Add boiling water and melt gelatin mixture. Stir gelatin mixture into berries. Add lemon juice. Chill for 1 hour. The berry mixture should be starting to set up and hold its shape, but should not be hardened all the way. Whip cream and mix in maple syrup and vanilla. Fold the whipped cream into the chilled berry mixture. Let set for twelve hours.

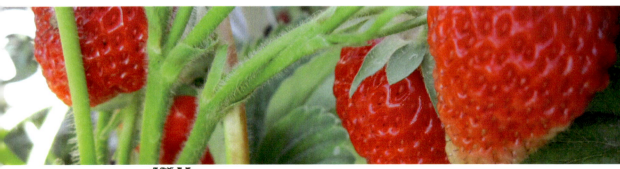

Grandma's Blueberry Pie Filling

Makes 1 pie

- 4 cups wild blueberries, fresh or frozen
- ¾ cup organic sugar
- 1 pinch of sea salt
- 4 tablespoons minute tapioca or arrowroot starch

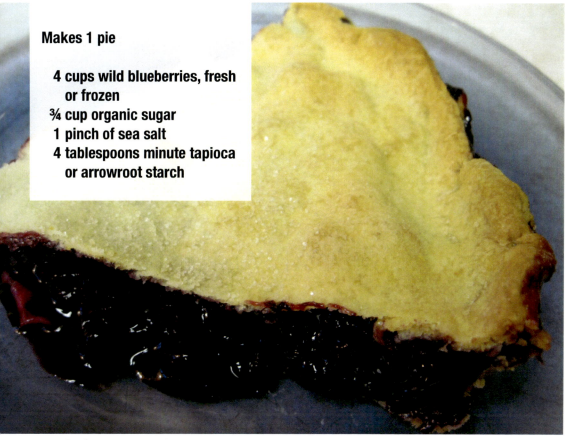

Preheat oven to 400°

Mix all ingredients in a bowl. Pour into a prepared pie crust (page 88). Cover with a second crust. Seal edges. Cut a few vent slots. Bake for 15 minutes. Reduce heat to 375° and bake for 45 minutes more.

Original recipe is from Sarah Katherine Maki.

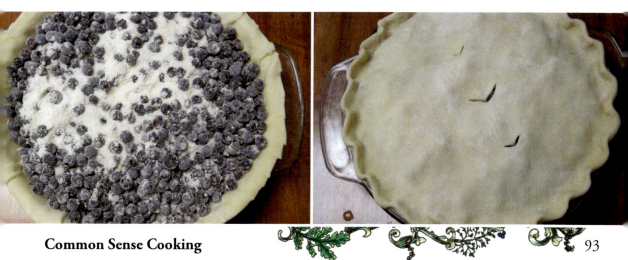

Zucchini Pie

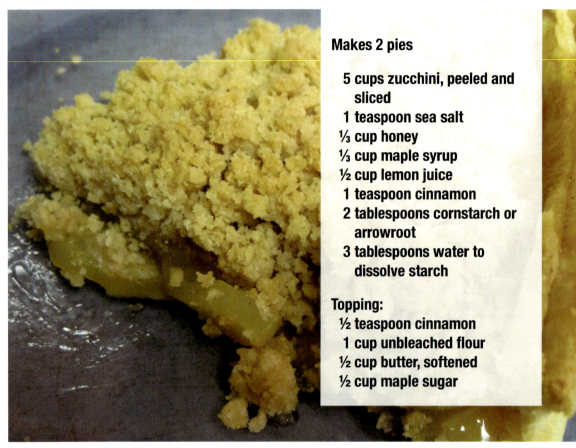

Makes 2 pies

- 5 cups zucchini, peeled and sliced
- 1 teaspoon sea salt
- ⅓ cup honey
- ⅓ cup maple syrup
- ½ cup lemon juice
- 1 teaspoon cinnamon
- 2 tablespoons cornstarch or arrowroot
- 3 tablespoons water to dissolve starch

Topping:
- ½ teaspoon cinnamon
- 1 cup unbleached flour
- ½ cup butter, softened
- ½ cup maple sugar

Preheat oven to 375°

Use pie crust recipe on page 90. Chill the dough while you make the filling. In a large saucepan, put the zucchini, salt, honey, maple syrup, lemon juice, and cinnamon. Bring to a boil. Reduce heat and simmer 20 minutes. Dissolve the cornstarch or arrowroot in 3 tablespoons water. Add to zucchini mixture and stir until thickened. Roll out crusts for 2 pie pans. Pour zucchini sauce into crusts. Mix cinnamon, flour, butter, and sugar until crumbly for topping. Top with topping. Bake for 30-35 minutes.

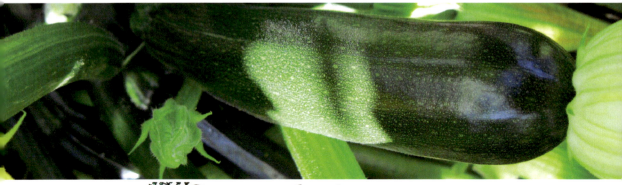

Rose Hip Sauce

Makes 1 quart

- 1 cup dry rose hips
- 1 quart water
- ⅓ cup honey
- 3 tablespoons arrowroot starch
- 1 tablespoon butter
- 1 teaspoon vanilla

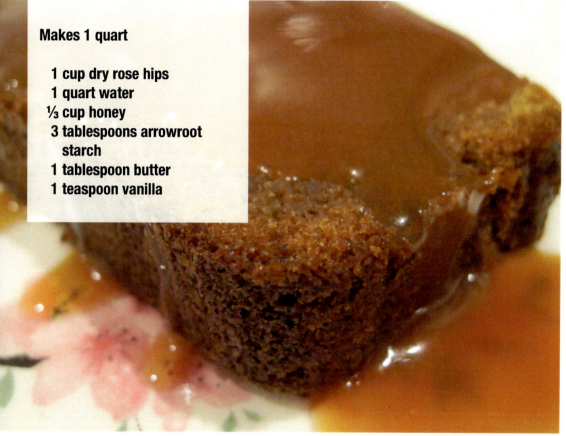

Measure rose hips into large bowl. Boil water and pour over rose hips. Cover and allow to stand for one hour. Strain off the tea liquid into a kettle, reserving ½ cup of the tea to melt the arrowroot. Add honey and heat to just below boiling. Dissolve arrowroot starch in reserved liquid. Stir into the heated brew. Continue stirring until sauce thickens and turns clear. Stir in butter and vanilla.

Serve either warm or cold with zucchini gingerbread (page 97) and whipped cream.

Rose hips can be purchased from places that sell bulk herbs and spices. Frontier Natural Products packages seedless cut and sifted rose hips.

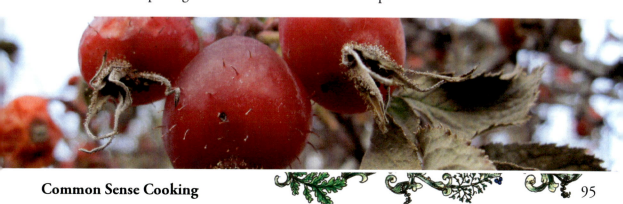

Zucchini Lemon Sauce

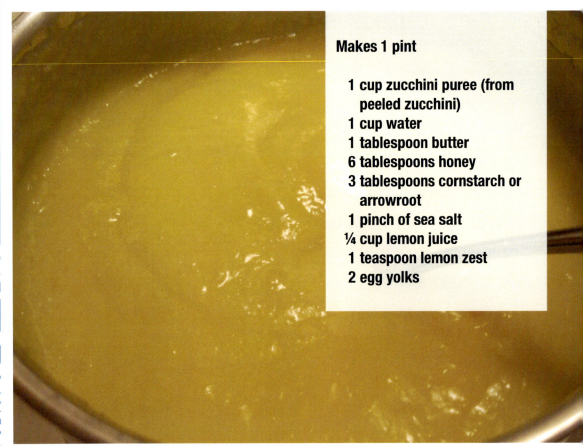

Makes 1 pint

- 1 cup zucchini puree (from peeled zucchini)
- 1 cup water
- 1 tablespoon butter
- 6 tablespoons honey
- 3 tablespoons cornstarch or arrowroot
- 1 pinch of sea salt
- ¼ cup lemon juice
- 1 teaspoon lemon zest
- 2 egg yolks

If you haven't already, peel and slice the zucchini. Cook in ½ cup of the water. Then puree it in a blender. Heat zucchini puree, butter, and honey in a saucepan. Bring to a boil. While it heats, combine cornstarch, rest of water, salt, lemon juice, and lemon zest. Stir to dissolve cornstarch. Add to zucchini mixture. Stir constantly until thick. In another bowl, beat egg yolks, and add a small amount of hot zucchini to the egg yolks. Stir well. Add more zucchini mixture, and stir again. Then add all the egg mixture back to the zucchini sauce. Cook about one minute more. Serve over zucchini gingerbread.

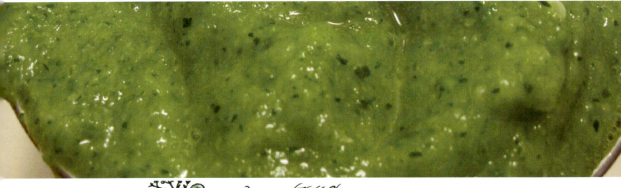

Zucchini Gingerbread

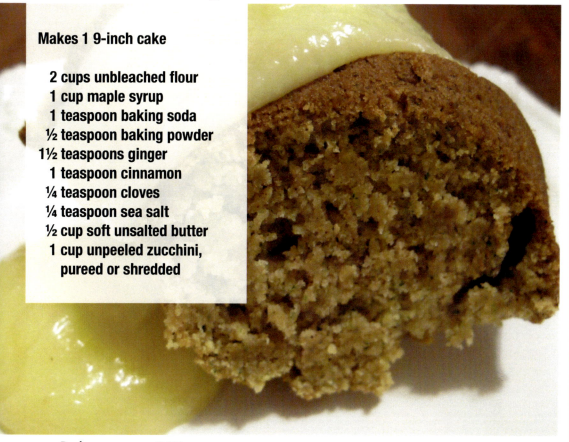

Makes 1 9-inch cake

- 2 cups unbleached flour
- 1 cup maple syrup
- 1 teaspoon baking soda
- ½ teaspoon baking powder
- 1½ teaspoons ginger
- 1 teaspoon cinnamon
- ¼ teaspoon cloves
- ¼ teaspoon sea salt
- ½ cup soft unsalted butter
- 1 cup unpeeled zucchini, pureed or shredded

Preheat oven to 350°

Measure all ingredients into large bowl of electric mixer. Mix at medium speed until well blended, about 2 minutes. Pour into a greased 9-inch cake pan. Bake for 30-40 minutes until cake springs back when touched lightly in center. Serve warm topped with lemon sauce (page 96), rose hip sauce (page 95), or applesauce and whipped cream. Double recipe for 9x13 or bundt pan.

Recipe works well even if substituting gluten-free flours.

Chocolate Chip Cookies

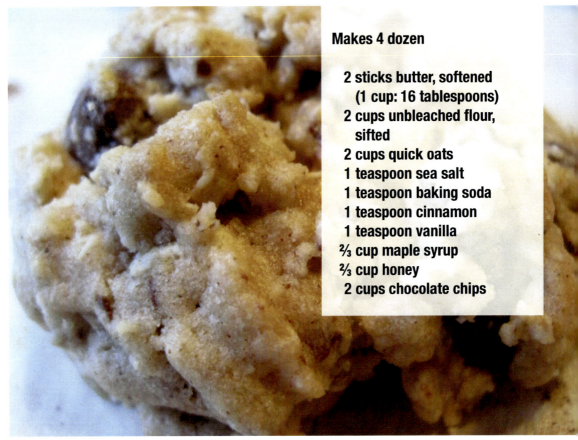

Makes 4 dozen

- 2 sticks butter, softened (1 cup: 16 tablespoons)
- 2 cups unbleached flour, sifted
- 2 cups quick oats
- 1 teaspoon sea salt
- 1 teaspoon baking soda
- 1 teaspoon cinnamon
- 1 teaspoon vanilla
- ⅔ cup maple syrup
- ⅔ cup honey
- 2 cups chocolate chips

Preheat oven to 350°
Combine all ingredients in a mixer except for the chocolate chips. Mix well. Then add chocolate chips and mix briefly. Scoop tablespoons of cookies onto a greased or parchment-lined baking sheet. Bake for 10-12 minutes until golden on top.

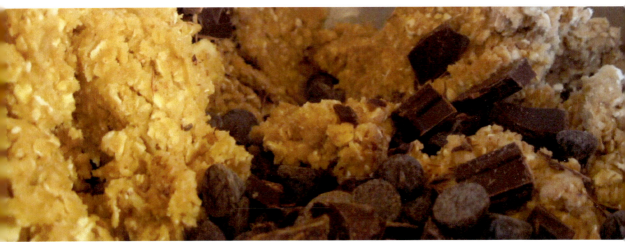

Spice of Life Specialty Foods PRESENTS

Cranberry White Chocolate Chip Cookies

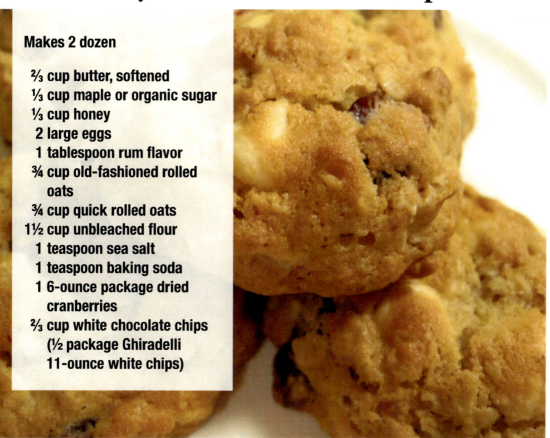

Makes 2 dozen

⅔ cup butter, softened
⅓ cup maple or organic sugar
⅓ cup honey
2 large eggs
1 tablespoon rum flavor
¾ cup old-fashioned rolled oats
¾ cup quick rolled oats
1½ cup unbleached flour
1 teaspoon sea salt
1 teaspoon baking soda
1 6-ounce package dried cranberries
⅔ cup white chocolate chips (½ package Ghiradelli 11-ounce white chips)

Preheat oven to 375°

Cream together butter, sugar, honey, eggs, and rum flavor. Dump the oats, flour, salt, and baking soda on top and mix lightly with a fork. Then mix into wet ingredients. Mix in the cranberries and white chocolate chips. Drop by cookie scoop or dessert spoon onto parchment lined cookie sheets. Bake 10-12 minutes or until golden brown.

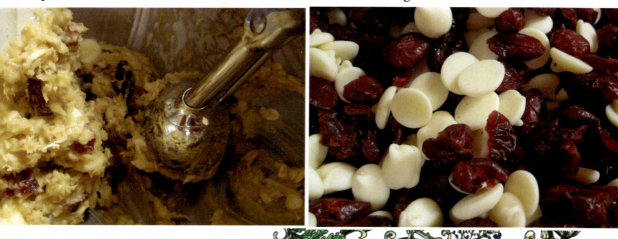

Common Sense Cooking

Finnish Cardamom Cookies

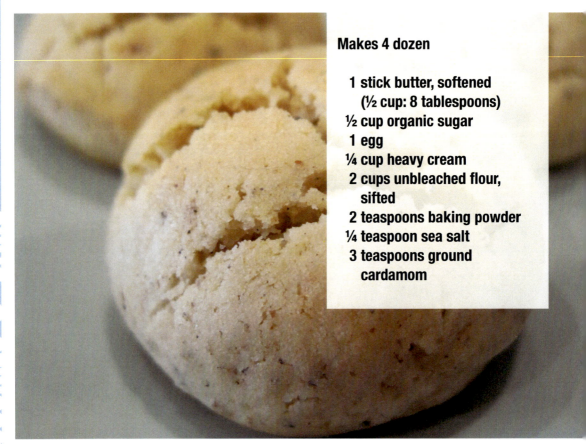

Makes 4 dozen

- 1 stick butter, softened (½ cup: 8 tablespoons)
- ½ cup organic sugar
- 1 egg
- ¼ cup heavy cream
- 2 cups unbleached flour, sifted
- 2 teaspoons baking powder
- ¼ teaspoon sea salt
- 3 teaspoons ground cardamom

Preheat oven to 375°

In mixer, cream butter and sugar together until light and fluffy. Then add the egg, beating until thick. Stir in the cream. In another bowl, mix flour, baking powder, salt, and ground cardamom. Add to liquid mixture. Mix until stiff dough forms. Chill for at least two hours. Shape chilled dough into small balls (1 inch in diameter or ½ ounce each) and arrange on baking sheet. Bake in hot oven for 10-12 minutes or until golden.

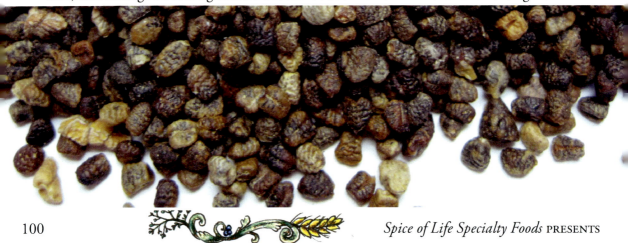

Spice of Life Specialty Foods **PRESENTS**

Cardamom White Caps

Makes 4½ dozen cookies

3½ cups unbleached flour
 1 teaspoon baking powder
 1 teaspoon ground cardamom
 ½ teaspoon sea salt
 ¾ cup unsalted butter, softened (1½ sticks)
 1 cup light brown sugar
   OR: ½ cup turbinado sugar & ½ cup maple sugar
 3 eggs
 1¼ teaspoons vanilla extract
 6 squares (1 ounce each) white chocolate
 1¾ cups walnuts, chopped

Glaze:
 1 cup powdered sugar
 3½ teaspoons milk

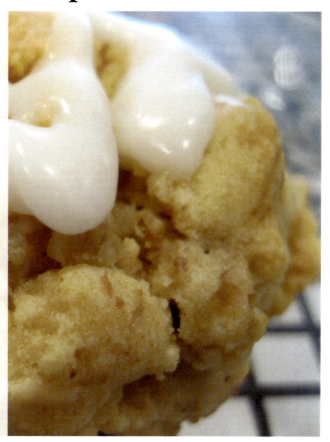

In a large bowl whisk flour, baking powder, cardamom, and salt. Set aside.

In another large bowl, beat butter for one minute. Add sugar and beat until smooth, about 2 minutes. Beat in eggs, one at a time. Beat in vanilla. Melt chocolate in microwave-safe bowl on high for one minute. Stir until smooth. Cool, then beat into mixture. Beat in flour mixture on low speed until just combined. Fold in chopped nuts. Cover dough; refrigerate for 2 hours.

Heat oven to 350° Drop dough in heaping tablespoons onto 2 ungreased baking sheets, about 12 cookies per sheet. Bake for 15 minutes or until set and lightly golden around edges. Mix powdered sugar and milk until smooth and consistency of honey. Drizzle over cookies when cool.

COOKIES & BARS

Common Sense Cooking

Ginger Snaps

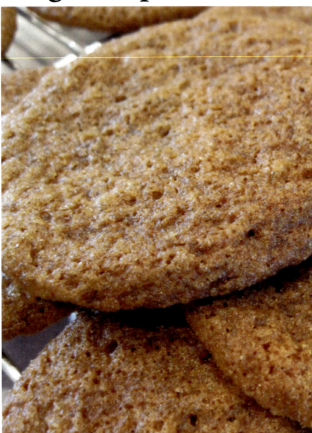

Makes about 50 cookies

- 2 cups unbleached flour, sifted
- 2 teaspoons baking soda
- 1 teaspoon cinnamon
- 1 teaspoon ginger
- ½ teaspoon sea salt
- ½ teaspoon ground cloves
- ¾ cup butter
- 3 tablespoons molasses
- 1 tablespoon honey
- 1 egg, beaten
- 1 cup organic sugar
- ⅓ cup candied ginger, minced (optional)

For dipping cookies:
- ½ cup organic sugar (raw sugar works well)

Preheat oven to 350°

Sift flour with baking soda, cinnamon, ginger, salt, and cloves. In a small bowl, mix butter, molasses, honey, egg and 1 cup sugar. In a large mixing bowl, mix candied ginger with flour mix. Gradually mix small bowl into the large bowl using your mixer. Chill dough for at least 1 hour. Put ½ cup sugar into bowl. Roll dough into 1 inch balls and roll in sugar. Bake for 8-10 minutes or until golden brown.

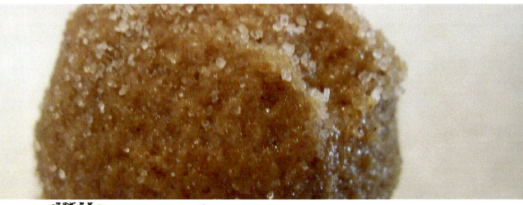

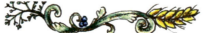

Spice of Life Specialty Foods PRESENTS

Finnish Ginger Cookies

Makes about 4 dozen 2 ½″ cookies

- ½ cup soft butter
- 3 cups unbleached flour
- 1 teaspoon baking powder
- ½ teaspoon sea salt
- 1 tablespoon cinnamon
- 1 tablespoon ground ginger
- ½ cup whipping cream
- ½ cup maple syrup
- ½ cup honey or brown sugar

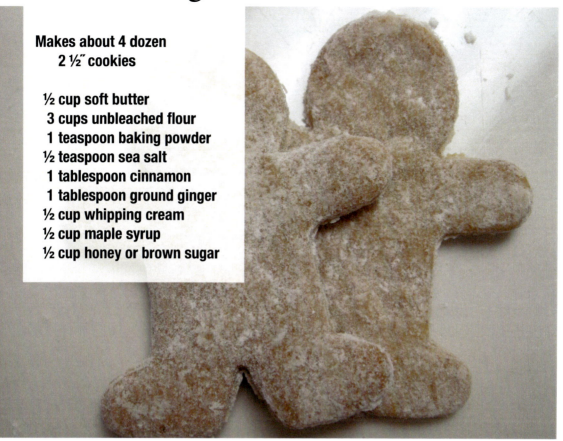

In food processor or mixer, mix butter, flour, baking powder, salt, cinnamon, and ginger. Then add cream, syrup, and honey and mix until smooth. Wrap dough in plastic wrap and chill.

Preheat oven to 375°

Take a half or third of the dough and roll out on a floured surface to about $\frac{1}{16}$ of an inch thick. Cut with cookie cutters. Place carefully on parchment-lined cookie sheets. Bake 7-10 minutes. This dough can also be cut and baked for a gingerbread house. The traditional shape for these cookies is round with a scalloped edge, but they are fun and tasty no matter what their shape.

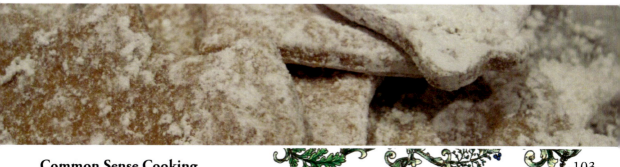

Pumpkin Cookies

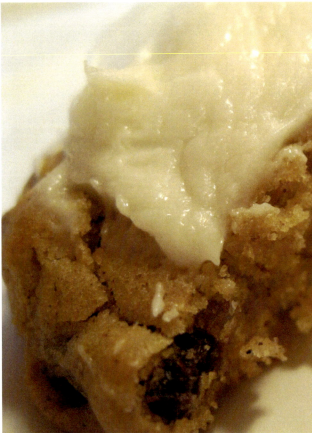

Makes about 2 dozen

  1 cup unbleached flour
  1 teaspoon baking powder
  ½ teaspoon baking soda
  ¼ teaspoon sea salt
  ½ teaspoon ginger
  ½ teaspoon cinnamon
  ½ teaspoon nutmeg
  ¼ teaspoon cloves
  2 eggs
  ½ cup organic sugar
  ½ cup maple sugar
  6 tablespoons butter, softened
  1 cup pumpkin or squash, cooked and pureed
  ½ teaspoon vanilla
  ½ cup walnuts, chopped
  ½ cup raisins

Frosting:
  4 ounces cream cheese warmed to room temperature
  ½ cup butter, softened
  3 cups powdered sugar
  ½ teaspoon vanilla

Preheat oven to 350°

Mix flour, baking powder, baking soda, salt, ginger, cinnamon, nutmeg, and cloves. Set aside. Beat eggs. Add organic and maple sugar and continue beating until light. Add 6 tablespoons butter and continue beating on high. Stir in pumpkin and ½ teaspoon vanilla. Fold in mixed dry ingredients. Add walnuts and raisins. Drop with scoop onto parchment. Bake for 13 minutes. Cool.

Mix cream cheese, ½ cup butter, powdered sugar, and ½ teaspoon vanilla. Frost cookies.

German Peppernuts

Makes about 5 dozen

- 4 cups unbleached flour, sifted
- 1 teaspoon baking soda
- ½ teaspoon sea salt
- 1 tablespoon cinnamon
- 1 teaspoon ground cloves
- 1 teaspoon nutmeg
- ¼ teaspoon black pepper
- 1 tablespoon ground cardamom
- 1 teaspoon ground anise seed
- ¼ pound candied orange peel
- ½ pound candied citron
- 2 tablespoons butter, softened
- 1 cup honey
- 5 eggs

Glaze
- 3 tablespoons milk
- 1½ cup powdered sugar

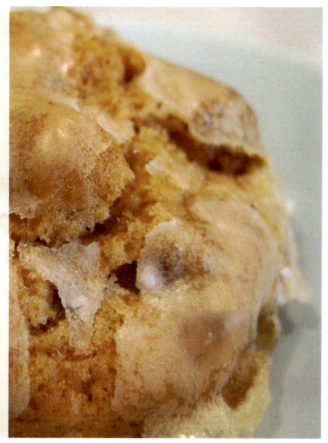

Mix together the flour, soda, salt, cinnamon, cloves, nutmeg, pepper, cardamom, and anise. Chop the orange peel and citron coarsely and add to the flour mixture. Add butter, honey, and eggs. Mix well. Chill dough for one hour. Then form into small balls the size of walnuts. Place on sheets of baking parchment cut to the size of cookie sheets. Let stand overnight uncovered at room temperature.

In the morning, preheat oven to 350°

Brush the cookies with glaze made from the milk and powdered sugar. Bake for 15 minutes.

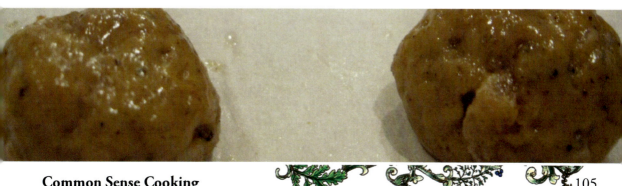

Macaroons

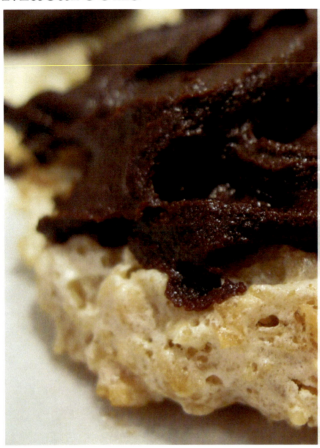

Makes 3 dozen

  3 egg whites
  ⅓ cup honey
  3 cups shredded
     unsweetened coconut
  2 teaspoons anise seed

Frosting:
  1 cup chocolate chips
  2-3 tablespoons half and half

Macaroons can be made in larger batches also:
  4 egg whites
  ½ cup honey
  4 cups shredded
     unsweetened coconut
  1 tablespoon anise seed

  6 egg whites
  ¾ cup honey
  6 cups shredded
     unsweetened coconut
  1 tablespoon anise seed

Preheat oven to 300°

Beat egg whites at top speed until stiff. Drizzle in honey while beating. Continue beating until very stiff peaks form. Measure coconut in another bowl. Grind anise seed and mix into coconut. Carefully fold coconut mixture into egg white mixture. Drop in heaping tablespoons onto greased or parchment papered baking sheet. Leave space between cookies, since they expand to about 2 ½ inches across. Bake for 30 minutes, but check after 20 minutes. The cookies should be starting to brown slightly.

Melt chocolate and cream on top of double boiler over medium heat or in a warm oven. Stir until smooth. Drizzle melted chocolate over cookies to form a cap on top. Let cool and harden. (For quicker cooling, put cookies on baking sheet and place briefly in freezer.) Some people prefer cookies unfrosted.

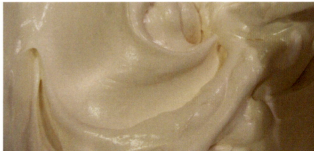

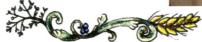

Spice of Life Specialty Foods PRESENTS

Pecan Tarts

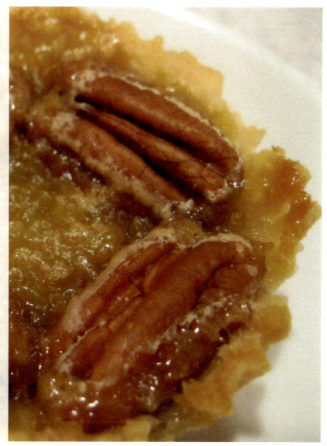

Makes 18 muffin-size tarts or about 4 dozen mini-muffin size tarts.

Crust:
  ½ cup butter, softened
     (1 stick: 8 tablespoons)
  ¼ cup maple syrup
  ½ teaspoon sea salt
  1½ cup unbleached flour, sifted

Filling:
  2 eggs
  1 cup maple syrup
  ½ teaspoon vanilla
  1 tablespoon unbleached flour
  4 tablespoons butter, melted
     (½ stick: ¼ cup)

72 pecan halves (4 for each muffin-size tart)

Preheat oven to 350°

Mix 1 stick softened butter, ¼ cup maple syrup, salt, and sifted flour together. Divide into 18 small balls. (Divide dough into 3 parts, each third into halves, and then each half into thirds again.) Line muffin pans with paper cups. Press each ball firmly into muffin pan using wooden tart tool or fingers. Make sure to press the dough up the sides forming cups (or shells) of dough. Blend eggs, 1 cup maple syrup, vanilla, 1 tablespoon flour, and ½ stick melted butter together. Pour this mixture into shells (about two tablespoons in each). Carefully place about four pecans on top of each. (Less for smaller tarts.) Bake for 20 minutes.

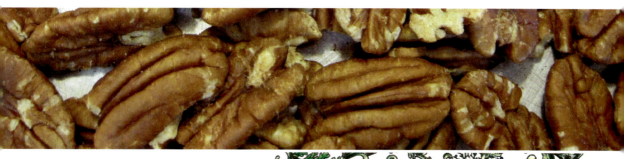

Common Sense Cooking

Granola Chews

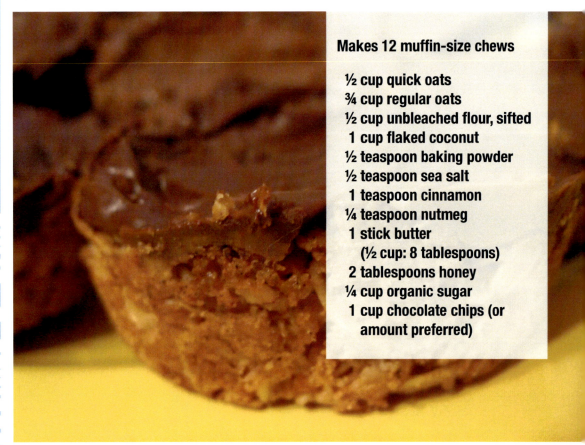

Makes 12 muffin-size chews

½ cup quick oats
¾ cup regular oats
½ cup unbleached flour, sifted
1 cup flaked coconut
½ teaspoon baking powder
½ teaspoon sea salt
1 teaspoon cinnamon
¼ teaspoon nutmeg
1 stick butter
   (½ cup: 8 tablespoons)
2 tablespoons honey
¼ cup organic sugar
1 cup chocolate chips (or amount preferred)

Preheat oven to 350°

Grease muffin tins. Mix oats, flour, coconut, baking powder, salt, cinnamon, and nutmeg together in a bowl. Melt butter in another bowl. When melted, add the honey and sugar. Stir well. Mix into dry ingredients. Divide mixture into 12 muffin tins and press down firmly. Bake for 9 minutes. Take out and sprinkle chocolate chips on top while still warm.

Optional: Once chocolate chips are melted, spread the chocolate.

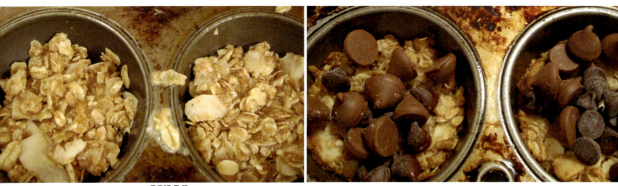

Spice of Life Specialty Foods PRESENTS

Chocolate Caramel Bars

Makes 18 bars in 9x13 pan

1¾ cups unbleached flour
1¾ cups quick oats
½ cup organic sugar
1 teaspoon sea salt
1 teaspoon baking soda
2½ sticks butter, softened: 10 seconds in microwave or until soft (1½ cups)
1½ cups chocolate chips
1 jar caramel topping (We prefer Mrs. Richardson's Butterscotch Caramel topping in 17-ounce jar.)

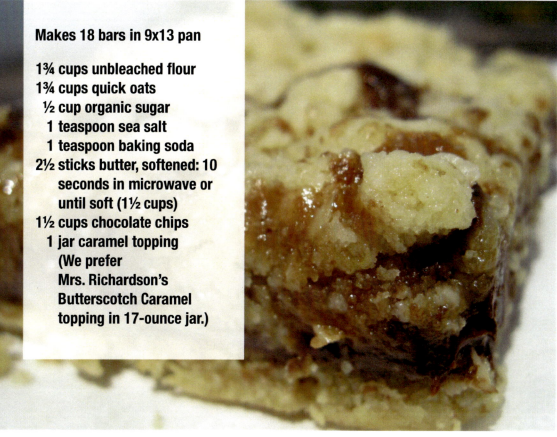

Preheat oven to 350°
   Mix flour, oats, sugar, salt, baking soda, and soft butter in a bowl until crumbly. Pat half of mixture into 9x13 pan. Bake for 9 minutes, then sprinkle chocolate chips over entire pan. Take a scraper and spread caramel topping over entire pan. Put rest of crumble mixture on top. Bake for 13 more minutes. Cool. Cut into 18 pieces.

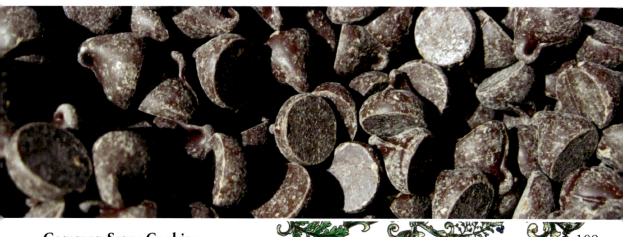

COOKIES & BARS

Blueberry Bars

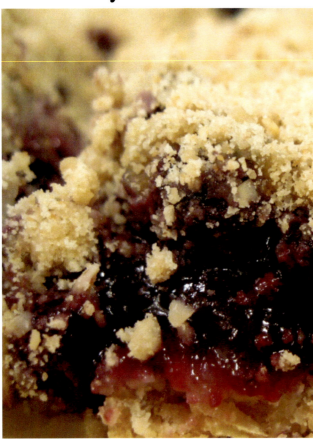

Makes 9 bars in 9x9 pan. Can double recipe for 18 bars in 9x13 pan.

¾ stick butter, softened (6 tablespoons)
⅓ cup maple sugar
1 cup unbleached flour, sifted
½ teaspoon sea salt
¼ teaspoon baking soda
½ cup quick oats
½ cup regular oats

Filling:
3 cups frozen blueberries
⅓ cup maple syrup
1 tablespoon cornstarch (melted in ½ cup water)
½ teaspoon butter
¼ teaspoon vanilla
1 sprinkle cinnamon

Preheat oven to 350°
    Mix butter, sugar, flour, salt, baking soda, and oats together until crumbly. Pat half of mixture into 9x9 pan. Put blueberries on crust. In saucepan, heat maple syrup and melted cornstarch until it thickens (should bubble or boil). Add butter and vanilla. Pour mixture over frozen blueberries. Sprinkle with cinnamon. Top with other half of crumble mixture. Bake for 45 minutes. Cut into 9 bars.

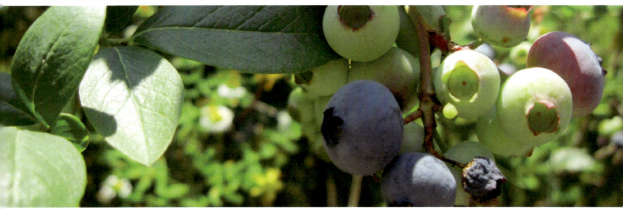

Spice of Life Specialty Foods PRESENTS

Apple Pastry

Makes 1 16x6 pastry

Crust:
 1 cup unbleached flour, sifted
 ⅛ teaspoon sea salt
 ¼ teaspoon baking powder
 1 tablespoon organic sugar
 ½ stick butter, softened
   (4 tablespoons: ¼ cup)
 ¼ cup cold milk

Filling:
 5 small to medium baking
   apples: peeled, cored, and
   sliced
 ¾ teaspoons cinnamon
 ¼ cup organic sugar

Glaze:
 ⅔ cup powdered sugar
 2 teaspoons milk
 ¼ teaspoon vanilla

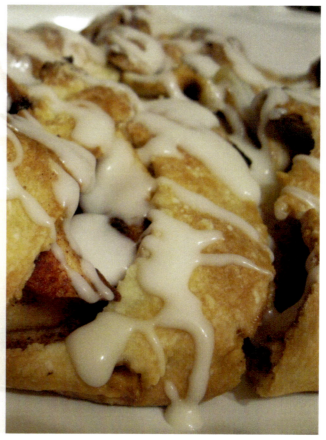

Preheat oven to 375°

Mix the flour with salt, baking powder, one tablespoon sugar, and butter until the mixture resembles fine crumbs. Add milk and stir with fork into a ball.

Roll dough on parchment to size of baking sheet (about 12x16). Arrange apples in center lengthwise. If the apples are too much, don't use them all. Sprinkle on sugar and cinnamon. Make slightly diagonal cuts about three inches long and one inch apart from the outside edge inward. Weave these strips over the top. Seal ends so filling doesn't run out. Bake for 45 minutes. Cool. Make glaze by combining powdered sugar, milk, and vanilla. Frost with glaze.

Chocolate Truffle

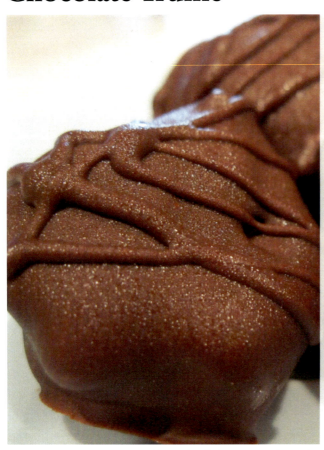

Makes about 20

- ¼ cup butter (4 tablespoons: ½ stick)
- 3 tablespoons cream
- ⅔ cup chocolate chips, OR 4 ounces chocolate baking bar, chopped
- 1 tablespoon flavoring of your choice, OR use one of the following:
- 2 teaspoons rum
- ¾ teaspoon butterscotch
- 10 drops of peppermint for filling and 3 drops in coating

Coating:
- ¾ cup chocolate chips
- 1½ tablespoons olive (or almond) oil

In a saucepan over medium-high heat, combine butter and cream. Bring to a boil and remove from heat. Stir in ⅔ cup of chocolate chips and flavoring. Stir until smooth. Chill until firm, about 2 hours.

Line a baking sheet with parchment or wax paper. Shape chilled truffle mixture by rounded teaspoons into small balls. Chill for about 30 minutes.

Put ¾ cup chocolate chips with olive oil in a glass bowl in microwave for 60 seconds or until smooth. Using two forks, dip each truffle into chocolate mixture and allow excess chocolate to drip back into bowl. Chill until set. Wrap with candy wrappers if you like.

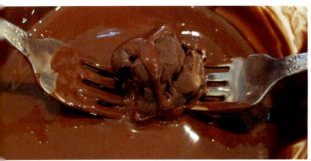
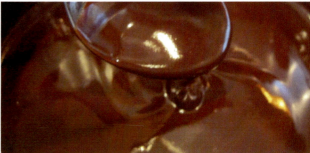

Spice of Life Specialty Foods **PRESENTS**

A GUIDE TO THE TRAVERSE CITY AREA
CRAFT BEER SCENE
AND
The People Behind It

By
Sue McVey

A Guide to the Traverse City Area Craft Beer Scene and the People Behind It
© 2017
Sue McVey

First Edition
Arbutus Press
PO Box 6450
Traverse City, Mi 49696
Info@arbutuspress.com

All rights reserved. No part of this book may be reproduced or transmitted in any form by any means, electronic, or mechanical, including photocopying and recording, or by any information storage and retrieval system, except for brief excerpts or by permission of the publisher.

ISBN 978-1-933926-54-4

Printed in the United States of America

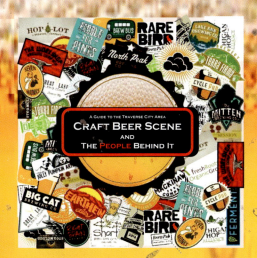

About the Book

The impetus for this book was developed over, of course, a delicious craft beer shared with fellow pickleball player and publisher, Susan Bays. The idea was to provide a guide to our local breweries with the intent of highlighting the people responsible for making our beer scene so awesome. For each brewery, taproom, supplier or activity, I interviewed the people featured in the book. The remaining content and photos were taken from their respective websites or Facebook pages.

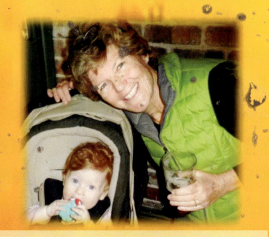

Two of my favorite things in the world, a pint of beer and my beautiful granddaughter.

About the Author

I'm a retired engineer who enjoys a good craft beer. I can't recall the first one I had, but it was years ago and I've enjoyed MANY since that day. I moved to Traverse City from Southern California ten years ago when there were only a few places serving craft brews. Now we are blessed with lots of good options.

I love to check out local brewpubs when I travel and I hope you can use this guide as a pub tour companion to help you navigate our area and discover some great craft beers!

Cheers!

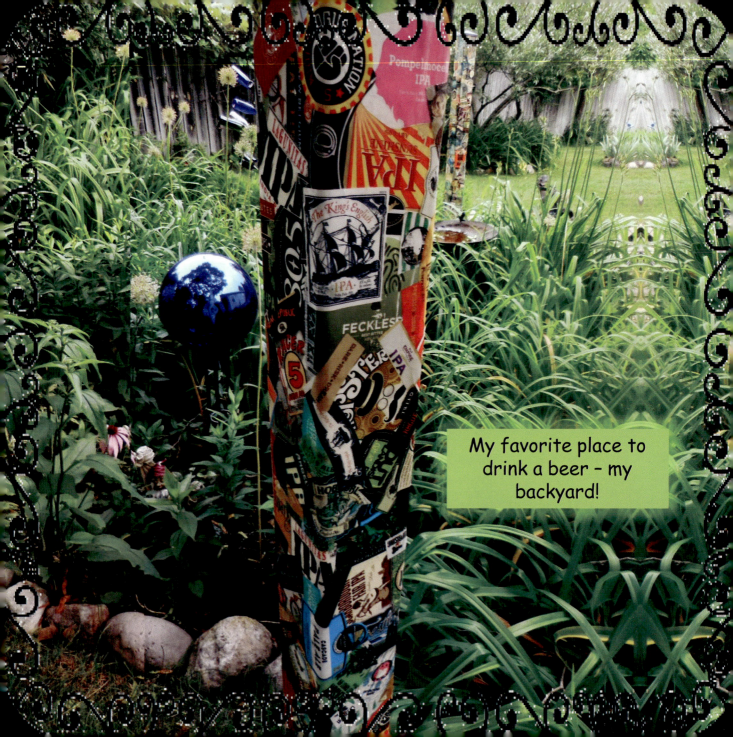

Contents

Featured Breweries / Head Brewer / Cicerone / Taproom Manager
    Big Cat Brewing / Aaron Ackley...10
    Brewery Ferment / Dustin Jones...14
    Brewery Terra Firma / John Niedermaier...18
    Earthen Ales / Jamie and Andrew Kidwell-Brix..22
    Hop Lot Brewing Company / Steve Lutke..26
    Jolly Pumpkin/Old Mission Brewing / Caleb Lentz.......................................30
    Lake Ann Brewing Co. / Matt Therrien..34
    Mackinaw Brewing / Mike Dwyer..38
    North Peak Brewing Company / Dave Hale..42
    Rare Bird Brewpub / Tina Schuett..46
    Right Brain Brewery / Russell Springsteen...50
    Seven Monks Taproom / Jason Kasdrof...54
    Short's Brewing Company / Tony Hansen..58
    Stormcloud Brewing / Brian Confer..62
    The Filling Station Microbrewery / Andy Largent..66
    The Mitten Brewing Co. / Dan Frank..70
    The Workshop Brewing Company / Michael Wooster..................................74

Featured Suppliers
    Fresh Roots Organic Growers / Joel Mulder...78
    Great Lakes Malting Co. / Jeff Malkiewicz...82
    Michigan Hop Alliance / Brian Tennis...86

Associated Activities
    TC Brew Bus / Troy Daly..91
    Kayak, Bike and Brew / Troy Daly..92
    Paddle for Pints / Troy Daly...94
    TC Cycle Pub / Kevin Farron..96
    Pour For More / Tina Schuett..98

Notes...100

Checklist..101

Maps
    Traverse City Area...102
    Traverse City...103

Meet the Featured Brewers

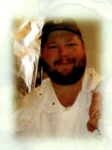

Big Cat Brewing
Aaron Ackley

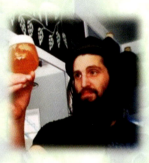

Brewery Ferment
Dustin Jones

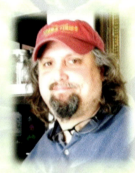

Brewery Terra Firma
John Niedermaier

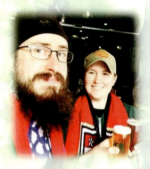

Earthen Ales
Jamie and Andrew Kidwell-Brix

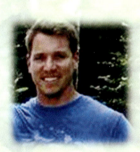

Hop Lot Brewing Co.
Steve Lutke

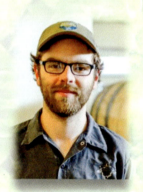

Old Mission Brewing
at Jolly Pumpkin
Caleb Lentz

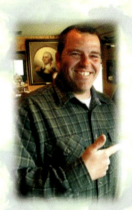

Lake Ann Brewing Co.
Matt Therrien

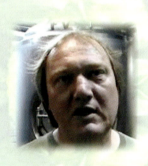

Mackinaw Brewing
Mike Dwyer

Meet the Featured Brewers

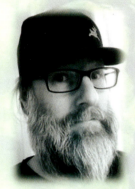
North Peak Brewing Co.
Dave Hale

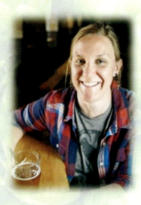
Rare Bird Brewpub
Tina Schuett

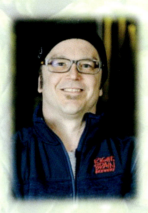
Right Brain Brewery
Russell Springsteen

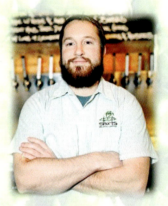
Short's Brewery Co.
Tony Hansen

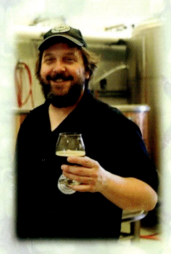
Stormcloud Brewing
Brian Confer

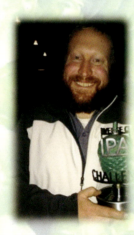
The Filling Station Microbrewery
Andy Largent

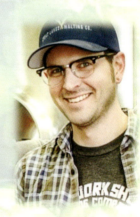
The Workshop Brewing Co.
Michael Wooster

Meet the:

Featured Taproom Managers

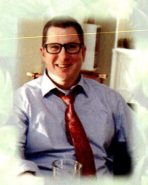
Seven Monks Taproom
Jason Kasdrof

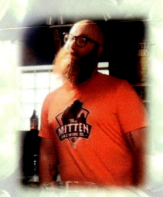
The Mitten Brewing Co.
Dan Frank

Featured Suppliers

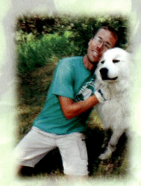
Fresh Roots Organic Growers
Joel Mulder

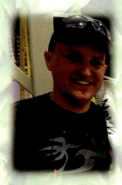
Great Lakes Malting Co.
Jeff Malkiewicz

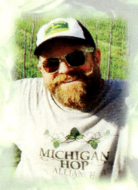
Michigan Hop Alliance
Brian Tennis

Activity Coordinators

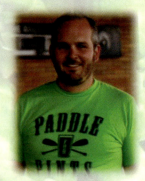
Paddle for Pints /
Kayak, Bike and Brew /
TC Brew Bus – Troy Daly

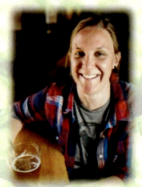
Pour For More
Tina Schuett

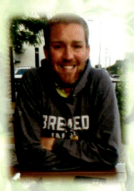
TC Cycle Pub
Kevin Farron

- For a quart of ale is a dish for a king. - **William Shakespeare**

- Beer – because no great story ever started with a salad. - **Anonymous**

- If God wanted us to drink filtered beer he wouldn't have given us a liver. - **Bell's Brewery motto**

- Buy a man a beer, and he wastes an hour. Teach a man to brew, and he wastes a lifetime. - **Charles Papazian,** American nuclear engineer, brewer and author

- Life's too short to drink cheap beer - **Anonymous**

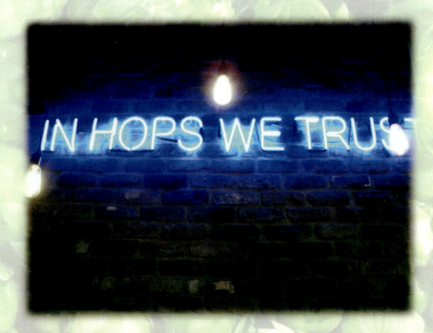

Big Cat Brewing

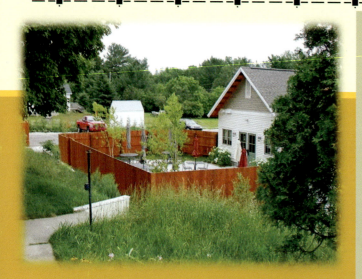

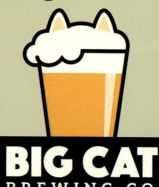

8699 S. Good Harbor Trail
Cedar
bigcatbrewing.com

We are Aaron and Nikki Ackley, owners, chef, brewer, waitress, bookkeeper, dishwashers, floor moppers.....you name it, we do it!

On May 27th, 2006 we opened as Cedar Rustic Inn. In 2012, Aaron started homebrewing. We had been craft brew fans for quite some time and it was exciting to watch and visit the breweries popping up around Traverse City. And out of a 5 gallon bucket, Aaron was making some good beer! Then, he got to thinking how much better the beer would be if only he had the proper equipment, and what a great addition the beer would be to our business! For two years, we scraped the money together and the commercial brewing equipment arrived in October 2014. We put our first beer on tap June 5, 2015, and Aaron has been a brewing maniac ever since.

The transition to Big Cat Brewing Company from Cedar Rustic Inn occurred March 1, 2016. It's a whole new adventure all over again! So, come on in and enjoy some great beer and food! We are open for breakfast, lunch and dinner. Specializing in American regional cuisine, or gourmet comfort food!

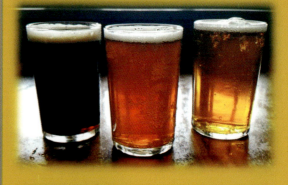

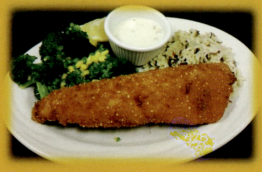

Head Brewer/Owner/Chef: Aaron Ackley

Background: "I started in the kitchen at age 18 and I've been at it for 28 years now. I had formal chef training in New York City at The Culinary Institute of America and received my Bachelor's degree in Restaurant Management. After finishing school I moved around to different settings and different jobs, including chef at hotels, a nursing home, country clubs and a management stint for Darden Restaurants. I am a Lansing native and eventually headed back to Michigan, settling in Cedar and working locally as a chef at The Homestead, Art's Tavern and Boone's. After Nikki and I got married, we opened a standard restaurant at our current location and I started home brewing. We hatched a plan to change our restaurant to a brewpub offering our own beer. I attended an intensive 8 day course in Vermont at the American Brewers Guild to help me transition to commercial brewing. It's been about 2 years now that we've had beer on tap. We keep increasing our equipment inventory, growing from the original 2 fermenters to 5 now to try and keep up with demand. The switch to brewpub included small tweaks to our menu, mostly the addition of a number of small plates. It's been fun to run a family business with my wife and two daughters. I like being my own boss and running my own show."

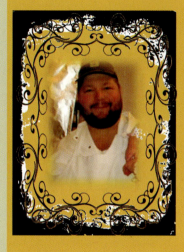

What motivates you? "I'm one of those guys that makes things. Some people are dreamers or problem-solvers, but I make things. My Mom was a sculptor so I grew up making things. Creating dishes, brewing beer, that's making things and that's me. I like to make things."

How do you decide what to brew? "I like to focus on what the customers want. IPAs and blondes are the most popular. I also need to keep in mind our food too. Our beer must be food-friendly."

How do you name your beers? "I've actually put up nameless beers before because we vacillate a lot with our naming. We try to be funny and clever. For example, when I named our **Lord Mutton Chops ESB**, I was envisioning a stodgy old Brit with big mutton chops and a monocle. Our **What's Hoppening IPA** was named one day when I was tossing around names in my head and I threw that one at my wife and she said, "not much". So it's kind of an on-going joke now to ask "What's Hoppening?"."

What were your original goals and have they changed? "Originally the idea came up as a kind of mid-life crisis. I was tired, stale. I started brewing at night in the restaurant kitchen and really enjoyed the brewing process. This led to our new direction. It's really helped me freshen up and be more engaged. I'm pretty happy with the current mix we have. We've developed a decent size catalog of beers now and I keep improving my brewing skills with every batch, starting with that first beer we brewed, a British Style IPA."

Big Cat Brewing – Aaron Ackley

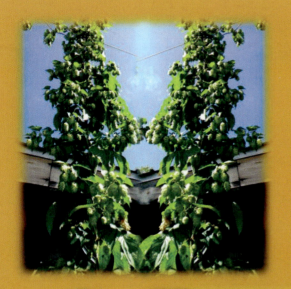

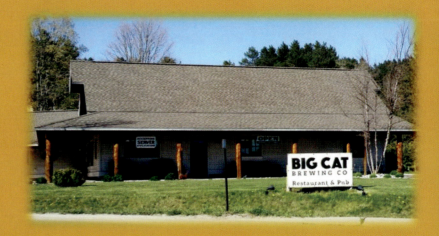

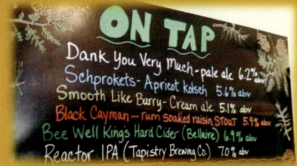

ON TAP
Dank You Very Much - pale ale 6.2% abv
Schprokets - Apricot kolsch 5.6% abv
Smooth Like Barry - Cream ale 5.1% abv
Black Cayman - rum soaked raisin Stout 5.9% abv
Bee Well King's Hard Cider (Bellaire) 6.9% abv
Reactor IPA (Tapistry Brewing Co.) 7.0% abv

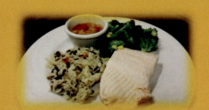

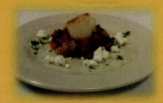

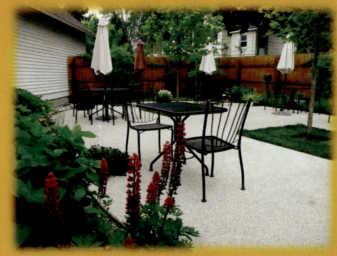

Big Cat Brewing – Aaron Ackley

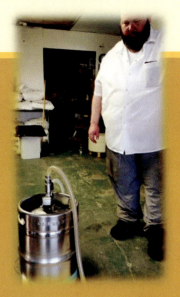

Fun fact: "I try to turn stress into humor. That's my survival trick. I make people smile and laugh. Humor fixes a lot of things."

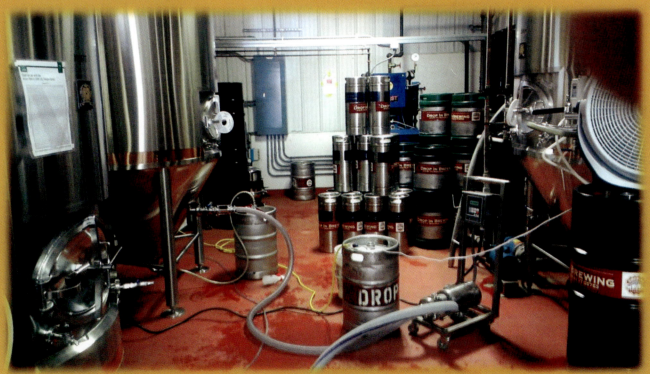

Brewery Ferment

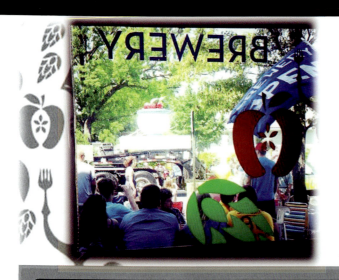

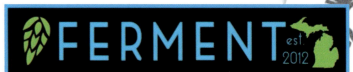

511 S Union Street
Traverse City
Breweryferment.com

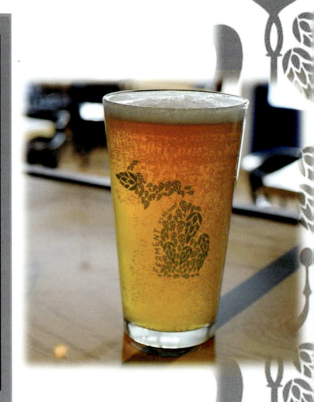

Ferment is an inviting, casual, neighborhood brewery that is truly all about the craft. Our unexpected styles and brewing techniques paired with local artisan handcrafted merchandise creates *The Ferment Experience* which cannot be found anywhere else. Come seek the unique!

We aim to make the most of what local growers have to offer, brewing with Northern Michigan ingredients as much as possible. We also have a small menu of unique bar snacks and outside food is welcome. We have five flagship beers on draft along with rotating specialties and bottled conditioned beers. Stop in, have a pint and you will notice the local difference.

Complimenting the libations and beer gear is a relaxed and fun atmosphere. We have dart boards, coloring books, playing cards, board games, and a TV for all your favorite sports.

Head Brewer: Dustin Jones

Background: "I was born and raised in Traverse City. I moved to Chicago after high school and I started home brewing. I liked to have friends over and do blind tastings with my beer vs. commercial beers. People consistently chose my beer. I decided to move back to Traverse with the intention of opening a brewery. I wanted it to be a small neighborhood spot where I would want to spend time – treat it like our living room. We try not to take ourselves too seriously. We try to have a range of beer styles on tap so we can educate people about craft beer."

What motivates you? "I'm a creative person. I like to draw influence from everywhere. I'm always in competition with myself to make better beer. I try to represent the area and what it means to so many people."

How do you decide what to brew? "We try to keep a mix on tap and bottled. There are lots of possibilities for creativity in this area with local ingredients - good water, hops, malt, and access to used barrels. I like to use different varieties of hops. I even do beers with no hops, ones that are very malt forward. We enjoy going to beer festivals and I always try to come up with unusual beers to bring."

How do you name your beers? "I get inspiration from lots of places – pop culture, good puns, or plays on words. For example, The **45th Parallale** and **Old Town Brown**. I like to have fun with the names, especially for the beers we bring to the festivals. I try to come up with something catchy so people will want to stop by our booth and give us a try."

What were your original goals and have they changed? "My goals are always changing. I've sacrificed a lot personally for this place. We're more focused now than ever. We love to do festivals and use them as a gauge of the landscape and what's happening with people and trends. We tend to listen to our customers more now than ever. I'm open to different types of business models to give people the experience we want them to have."

Brewery Ferment – Dustin Jones

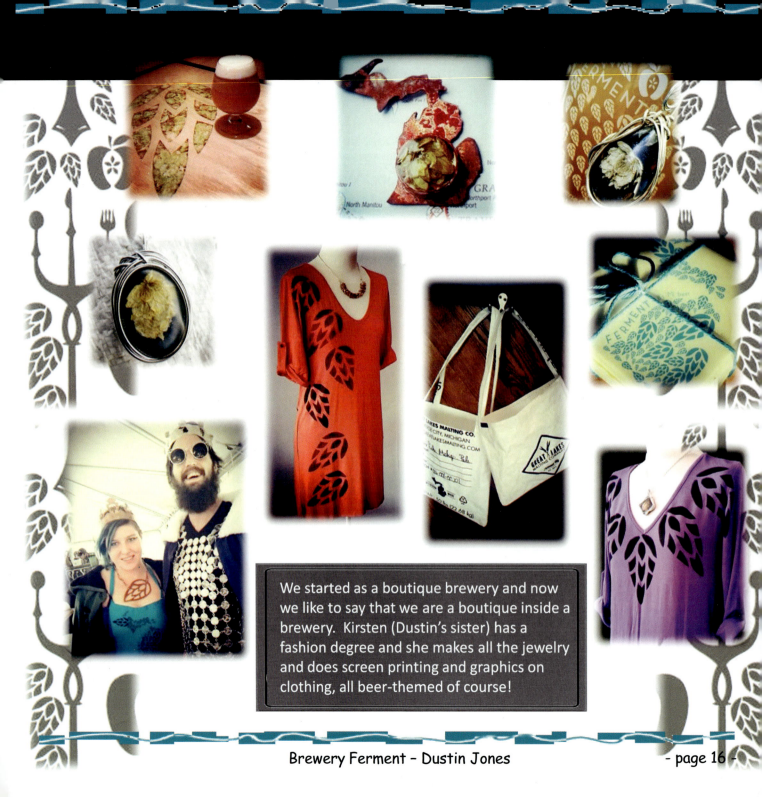

We started as a boutique brewery and now we like to say that we are a boutique inside a brewery. Kirsten (Dustin's sister) has a fashion degree and she makes all the jewelry and does screen printing and graphics on clothing, all beer-themed of course!

Brewery Ferment – Dustin Jones

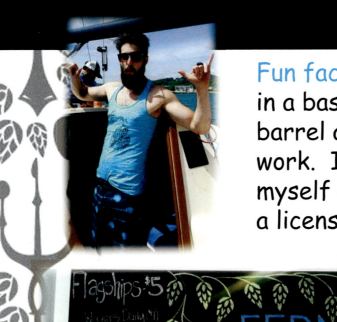

Fun fact: "I'm just a maniac in a basement brewing one barrel at a time and making it work. I like to refer to myself as a homebrewer with a license."

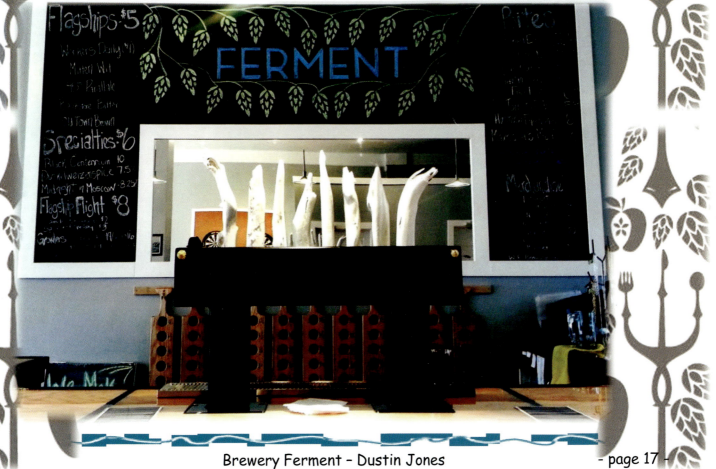

Brewery Ferment – Dustin Jones

Brewery Terra Firma

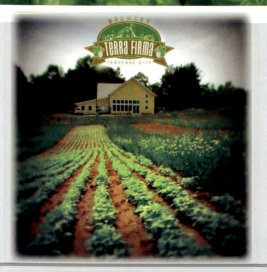

2959 Hartman Road
Traverse City
Breweryterrafirma.com

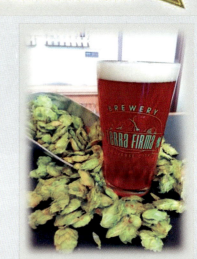

Brewery Terra Firma is a production brewery, tap room, and MAEAP certified farm located on 10 acres in Traverse City, Michigan. We produce delicious, culinary-inspired beers using sustainable methods, including an innovative water capture system in our brew house that has allowed us to reclaim over **185,000 gallons of water** from the manufacturing process for reuse as irrigation and fertilization on our farm crops. The other major opportunity for conservation that we identified was the capture and reuse of "waste" heat. Excess heat from the brewing process is harvested and used to heat water for cleaning the equipment at the end of the day, and also used to preheat water for the next brew. Heat from fermentation and refrigeration is captured via a heat pump and heat exchanger, and then sent through the in-floor heating system in our taproom during the cooler months. Through most of the fall, winter and spring, we're able to keep our taproom nice and toasty on reclaimed heat alone!

Stop by our taproom at 2959 Hartman Road in Traverse City to sample our beers, or find us throughout Michigan at your favorite bar or restaurant. We have locally-made snacks and sodas available for purchase, or bring along a meal from your favorite eatery and enjoy a tasty Brewery Terra Firma beer with it.

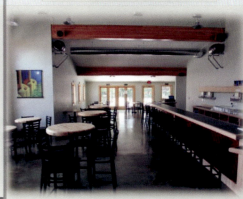

Head Brewer / Owner: John Niedermaier

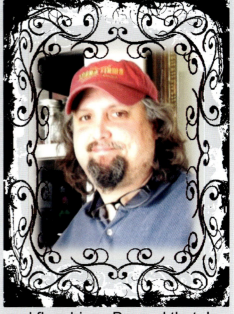

Background: "I was born and raised in Traverse City and I got into cooking over 25 years ago. That led to home brewing and eventually a full time commercial brewing job at Traverse Brewing Company (the first brewery in the Traverse City area). At Traverse we used to put grains out back in the garden as mulch. This spawned the idea of finding more ways to eliminate waste and be more efficient. That's where the idea behind Brewery Terra Firma came from. It took awhile to find the right property, though, and really get started."

What motivates you? "I love using the same non-traditional ingredients in both cooking and brewing. For example, we brew a beet beer which pairs well with salads and seafood and has been used as the base of a glaze served over pork belly at one of our beer dinners at Cook's House."

How do you decide what to brew? "We have our standard year-round flagships. Beyond that, I like to listen to our customers to see what they'd like to see brewed. I have over 1,000 recipes for all different types of beer. We also like to brew beers we haven't done lately as well as seasonal beers made with local ingredients. Our goal isn't just to be sustainable. We also want to support local farmers and encourage growing a community."

How do you name your beers? "They all have stories. I try to make sure they all mean something and I pretty much name all the beers myself. There are a few I haven't named, but not many."

What were your original goals and have they changed? "My original goal was to produce a huge variety of stylistic and non-stylistic beers. I love the freshness of the product and the closer you live to the brewery the better tasting the beer. So I wanted lots of styles done well so I could live in that magical world where I was surrounded by fresh beers. This goal hasn't really changed much over the years. At times, the popularity of some beers does keep me from brewing everything I would otherwise choose to brew."

Awards and Distinctions

- Michigan's first agricultural brewery
- Traverse City's only brewery not on the waste stream
- Traverse City's only brewery with it's own well
- John won multiple gold, silver and bronze medals at the World Beer Expo over the years when he was at Traverse Brewing.

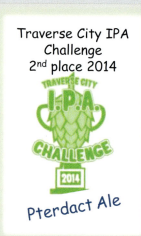

Traverse City IPA Challenge 2nd place 2014

Pterdact Ale

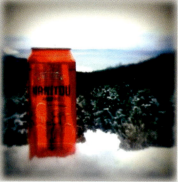

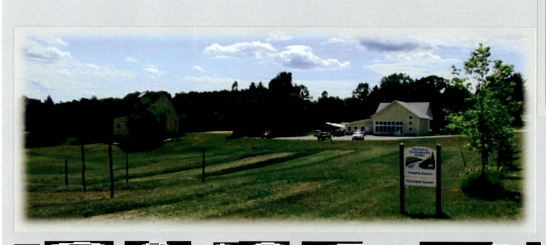

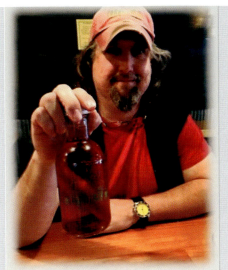

Fun fact: "I love really crappy Sci-Fi films like Attack of the Crab Monsters and Attack of the Puppet People. I like to call them 'craptastic'."

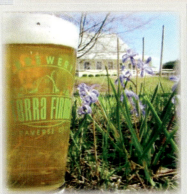
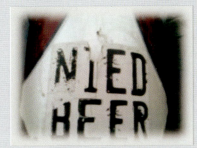
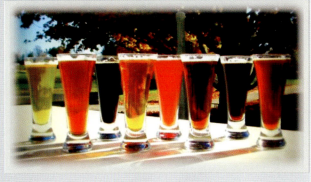
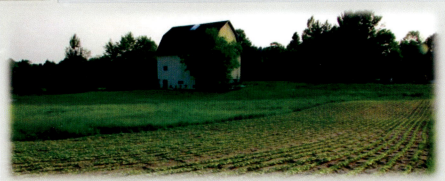

Earthen Ales

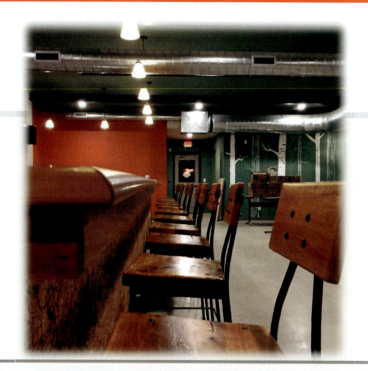

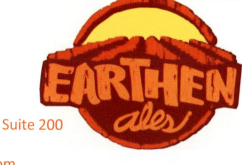

1371 Gray Dr., Suite 200
Traverse City
earthenales.com

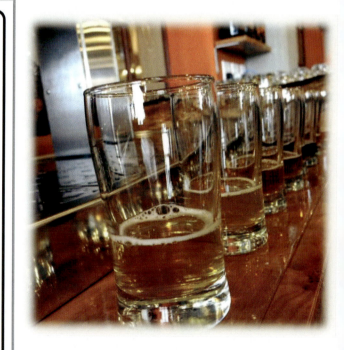

What happens when two brewers fall in love? This is what happens: you start by brewing more beer than you know what to do with. Then you move on to talking about quitting your day jobs and opening your own brewery together. And then, if you're lucky, that's what actually happens.

We are Jamie and Andrew Kidwell-Brix, and we like to make beer. No, seriously. We really like to make beer, so we were making more than we could drink ourselves. So we invited over our friends, and still we had too much beer, so we decided we needed more friends, and that is where you come in. We opened Earthen Ales to share our beer with you, dear reader.

What kind of beer do we make? We like to brew beer that reminds us of places we've lived, places we've visited, and the friends we've made along the way. More importantly, we like to brew beer that brings people together here in beautiful Northern Michigan.

Earthen Ales – Jamie and Andrew Kidwell-Brix

Head Brewers/Owners:
Jamie and Andrew Kidwell-Brix

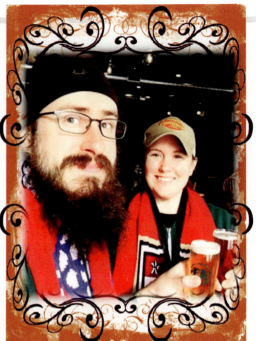

Background: **Jamie**: "We are very much a team. We had both brewed before we met and once we started brewing together it got out of control! I love collaborating with Andrew and our new brewery is a fun venture together."
Andrew: "We brewed our first batch of beer together at a friend's house with borrowed equipment and we've only gotten more interested. It's been the good kind of rabbit hole."

What **motivates** you? **Andrew**: "I enjoy making people happy by handing them a pint of my beer and watching them smile and laugh."
Jamie: "I want to serve beer with a sense of place and community and share that with patrons, friends and family."

How do you decide **what to brew**? **Jamie**: "I draw inspiration from different experiences or places we've been. For example, our *Lime Wit* reminds me of the south and growing up. I'm also interested in historical styles and reimagining them into something more modern."
Andrew: "We mostly brew things we want to drink. The point of germination varies based on place or memory or sometimes new ingredients or new techniques."

How do you **name your beers**? **Andrew**: "I like simple names like *Sweetbrier Wheat* that invoke memories like sunshine and fruit and picking berries in Northport on a summer afternoon."
Jamie: "We are simple folk. We tend to name the beers what they are. If you look at the name you know what you're gonna get."

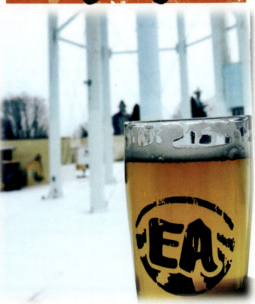

What were your original goals and have they changed? Jamie: "We have only been open a few months so far and our goal is to make good beer. Beyond the pint, beyond the beer we want to be a community space where people can come together."

Andrew: "We want to have happy people enjoying our beer and having a good time. Our reward is having people enjoy our beer and we hope to make a living off that!"

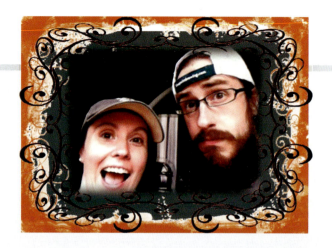

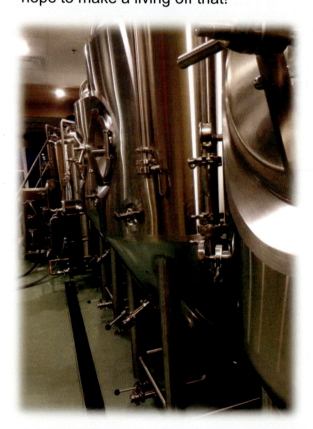

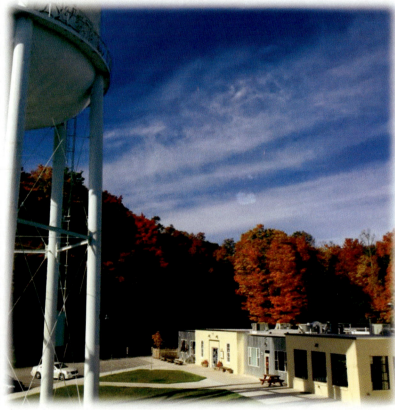

Earthen Ales – Jamie and Andrew Kidwell-Brix

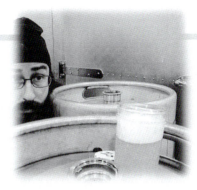

Fun fact: Andrew had a brief stint as a farmer growing vegetables and raising animals on a friend's farm in Northport.

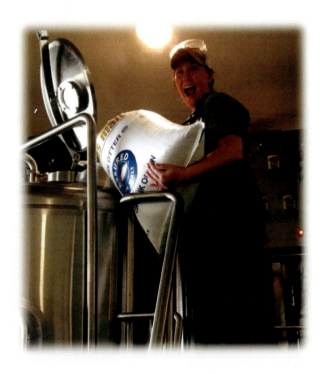

Fun fact: Jamie is a former local government urban planner and self-proclaimed "big nerd". She can spend hours chatting about the topic of how beer relates to cities and communities.

Hop Lot Brewing Company

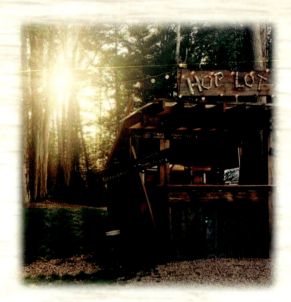

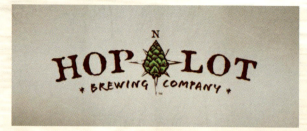

658 S. West-Bay Shore Drive
Suttons Bay
hoplotbrewing.com

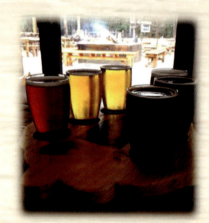

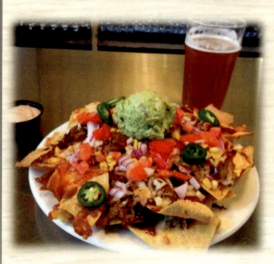

Originally from Holland, MI then later residing in Chicago, it was time for us to journey back to Michigan and create a very unique four-seasons Microbrewery and Beer Garden in beautiful Northern Michigan. With family ties to Suttons Bay, it was the perfect location to both embrace the local beer culture while also embracing the outdoors. We're two brothers with a passion for consistent and fresh-tasting craft beer.

What you can expect at the brewery
- Knowledgeable, welcoming, and friendly staff.
- Consistent and fresh-tasting craft beer year-round at our taproom.
- One-of-a-kind outdoor beer garden with an 'Up North' twist for your drinking pleasure.
- On-site hop garden.
- 10-14 taps with main stays and rotating taps.
- Not just "hoppy" beers. Although it's in our name, we brew all styles of beer, for all different tastes.

Head Brewer / Co-founder: Steve Lutke

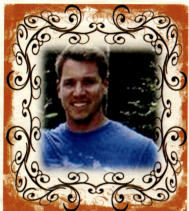

Background: "I started out as a home brewer in a Chicago apartment. Since I have a pre-med degree, I am really interested in the science of brewing. I am a graduate of the Siebel Institute of Technology with an Associates in Brewing Technology. I designed and built my own home brew system for my apartment and started tinkering with recipes. At one point, I had over 900 bottles of beer in the apartment! I brewed the beer for my wedding reception and there were some key people in attendance that liked my beer and encouraged me to seriously consider a beer career. My new wife and I ended up moving to Sutton's Bay and were planning a brewery in the agricultural district along with a hop farm, but the zoning laws didn't allow breweries at the time. Meanwhile, we looked around at property and found our current location, shifted gears and decided to open a brewery. My brother, Drew, runs the front of the house and my wife, Sarah, takes care of the finances.

What **motivates** you? "I like refining the process. For me, it's a big experiment. Each time I brew I try to hone the craft and I am constantly trying to improve the product."

How do you decide **what to brew?** "There are a number of factors that determine what we brew. I don't necessarily like to follow trends, although a lot is decided by the customers. Their demand sets a direction for styles. New hop varieties may come along that lead to a beer choice. There's always our mainstays that need brewing and with summer approaching, there's the challenge of creating lighter beers with our twist."

How do you **name your beers?** "Most of our original beers are named for inside jokes from our construction phase – like **Roughsawn Wood** or **Tippy Canoe**. Some names come from my Uncle. For example, he runs a highway fruit stand that we tease him is overpriced, hence the name **Highway Robbery**. We like to use funny sayings that mean something. Once we spent hours trying to name a beer and someone noted, "What a Wasted Effort", and **Wasted Effort** was born!"

What were your original goals and have they changed? "Originally, we just wanted to survive and make consistently good product. We had no plans for a kitchen. Now we're adding a kitchen expansion and we upgraded our brew system from the original 3 barrels to our current 10 barrels. We plan to stay in-house, though. We want to focus on quality product and improving the overall experience at Hop Lot."

Awards and Recognition

Mlive – Best New Brewery in Michigan opened in 2014 - 2016
4th place

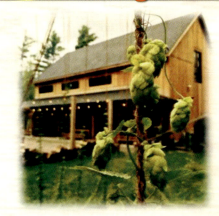

MyNorth/Traverse Magazine
Red Hot Best 2017
- Best Spot for Live Music – 1st place
- Best Outdoor Dining – 2nd place
- Best Brewer – 3rd place
- Best Local Brewpub or Taproom – 3rd place

Red Hot Best 2016
- Best New Restaurant – 3rd place

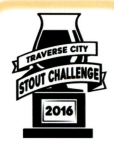

2nd place - Inaugural Traverse City Stout Challenge
Leelanau Exchange

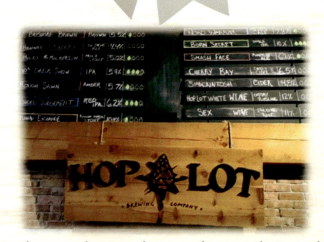

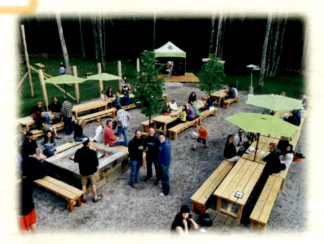

Hop Lot Brewing – Steve Lutke

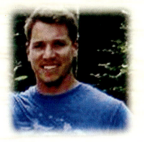

Fun fact: "I am the current president of the Village of Sutton's Bay."

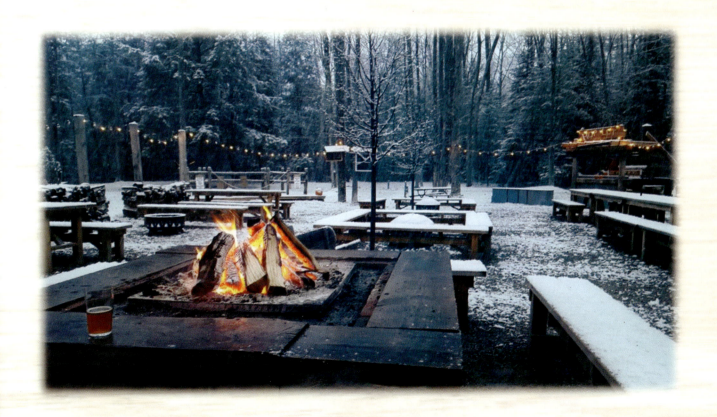

Old Mission Brewing at Jolly Pumpkin

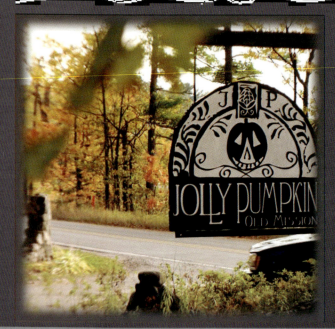

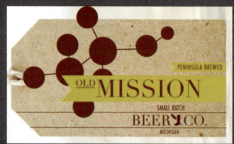

13512 Peninsula Drive
Old Mission Peninsula
Traverse City
jollypumpkin.com

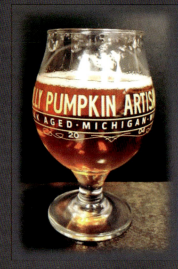

Old Mission Brewing's home is on-site at Jolly Pumpkin on the Old Mission Peninsula. Beers brewed at Old Mission Brewing as well as Jolly Pumpkin Artisan Ales, headquartered in Dexter, Michigan, are under the umbrella of Northern United Brewing Company and beers from both breweries are served at Jolly Pumpkin on Old Mission.

Inspired by natural surroundings, the esteemed Jolly Pumpkin Restaurant, Microbrewery & Distillery offers a rustic atmosphere marked by fireside warmth and earthy woods in a comfortable cottage-like setting. Stop in for lunch or dinner to enjoy delectable American fare, as well as a full lineup of craft beers and spirits.

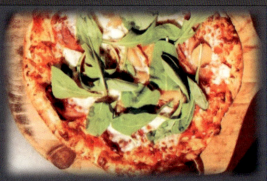

Old Mission Brewing at Jolly Pumpkin – Caleb Lentz

Old Mission Brewing Head Brewer: Caleb Lentz

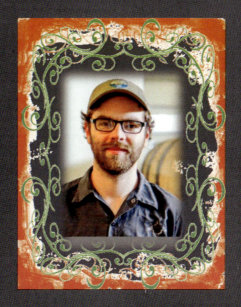

Background: Caleb is a Traverse City native who joined AmeriCorps out of college and did conservation work downstate for a year. After that stint he returned to Traverse City. He was a home brewer and landed a part-time job brewing at Jolly Pumpkin. He returned to school at Northwestern Michigan College and continued to work at Jolly Pumpkin where he's now worked his way up to head brewer!

What **motivates** you? "I like the idea of creating something for others to enjoy. It's a really fulfilling feeling to have someone say they enjoy my beer. Putting joy into someone else reinforces that all the hard work is worth it. I also enjoy the sense of community amongst our local brewers. We are competitive, yet friendly. We like to help each other push the envelope and we advocate for each other."

How do you decide **what to brew**? "Seasons are a heavy influence for us. The themes of our beers are centered around the Old Mission Peninsula and adhering to ingredients available from local farms. We used local organic Montmorency cherries in our recently released Chocolate Cherry Stout. We also use lots of local hops."

How do you **name your beers**? "I usually stick with the Old Mission theme and geographic locations or history of the peninsula. ***Postmaster Stone Brown Ale*** is named after the first postmaster and ***Pratt's Pale Ale*** is named for the first lighthouse keeper."

What were your original goals and have they changed? "My original goal was to study freshwater sciences, but when I got the job as a part time brewer while in school at NMC I loved it and decided to change careers to becoming a brewer."

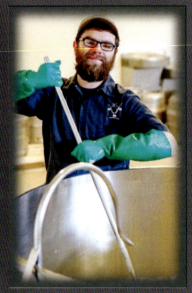

Fun fact: Caleb was born without wisdom teeth.

Fun fact: Evan is fluent in Norwegian.

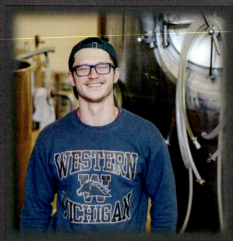

Assistant Brewer: Evan Spaulding

Head Brewer: Caleb Lentz

Co-Founder / Master Brewer: Mike Hall

Master Brewer Mike Hall is the big gun on Old Mission Peninsula. A native of Nova Scotia, Mike is ultimately responsible for the sublime list of beers and spirits at Northern United Brewing Company.

Mike is a world-renowned brewer, designer and educator. He was elected a Senior Member in the International Brewers Guild. Before becoming a partner in Northern United Brewing Company, Mike trained more than 100 brewers. He has participated in the design, building, installation and/or start up of over 50 breweries and distilleries around the globe, from as far away as Siberia to the Bahamas and several right here in Michigan. As managing partner of Northern United Brewing Company, Mike enjoys collaborating with both Old Mission head brewer, Caleb Lentz, as well as Jolly Pumpkin Artisan Ales head brewer, Ron Jeffries. Between Mike and Ron they have over 50 years of brewing experience and time at internationally renowned breweries such as Dogfish Head and Jolly Pumpkin, meaning drinkers can rest assured that the brews offered are of the utmost quality.

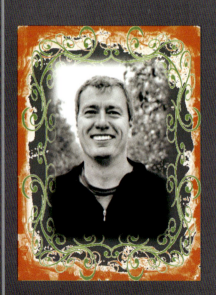

Old Mission Brewing at Jolly Pumpkin - Caleb Lentz

Also served at Jolly Pumpkin are Jolly Pumpkin Artisan Ales which are brewed in Dexter Michigan by head brewer Ron Jeffries

Jolly Pumpkin beers are known the world over. Crafted with French and Belgian yeasts in open fermentation vessels then conditioned for months in oak casks, these internationally acclaimed beers are unforgettable for their truly unique flavors and depth of character. Sweet. Sour. Satisfying.

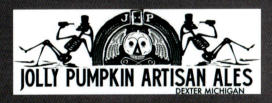

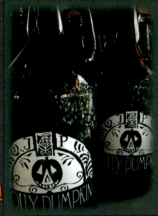

Jolly Pumpkin Artisan Ales Awards and Recognition

Bam Bière
- Great American Beer Festival Bronze in 2005
- Men's Journal Choice as one of the Top 25 beers in America

Oro de Calabaza
- Great American Beer Festival Gold Medal in 2004
- Great American Beer Festival Bronze in 2005
- Rated #1 Belgian Golden Ale by The New York Times in 2010

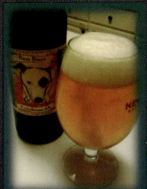

Style: Saison/Golden Farmhouse Ale
ABV: 4.5% **IBUs:** 25
Available: Year Round
Naturally cloudy and dry hopped for a perfectly refreshing balance of spicy malts, hops and yeast.

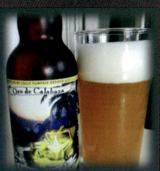

Style: Artisan Wild Ale
ABV: 8% **IBUs:** 30
Available: Year Round
Brewed in the Franco-Belgian tradition of strong golden ales. Spicy and peppery with a gentle hop bouquet and beguiling influence of wild yeast.

Lake Ann Brewing Co.

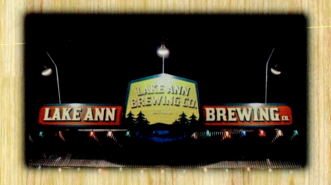

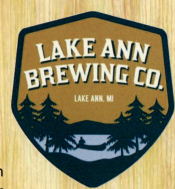

6535 First Street
Downtown Lake Ann
lakeannbrewing.com
(231) 640-2327

Lake Ann Brewing Company specializes in craft beers as well as local ciders, mead, and wine. A casual, rustic "up north" tavern with a large outdoor patio, open weather permitting. Live music on Tuesdays year-round. Music on the patio during the summer months Tuesday-Saturday (weather permitting). Full food menu from The Stone Oven restaurant right next door. "Great beer without the pomp and circumstance."

The work began in March 2014. With the help of family, friends and talented craftsmen from the areas surrounding L.A., we were able to transform the long neglected, bank-owned, L.A. Cafe (a tear down in many people's eyes) into Lake Ann Brewing Company. The vision for the building was to create a spot where neighbors, friends, and visitors alike could enjoy a fine libation, not take anything too seriously and learn more about the people and the history that make Lake Ann special.

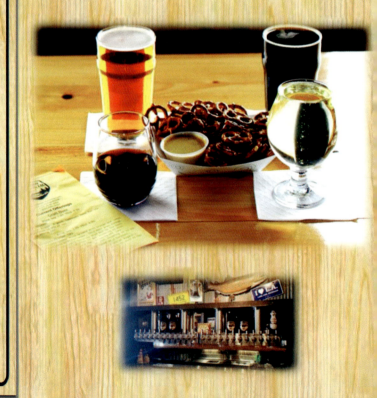

Lake Ann Brewing Co. – Matt Therrien

Co-Owner / Head Brewer: Matt Therrien

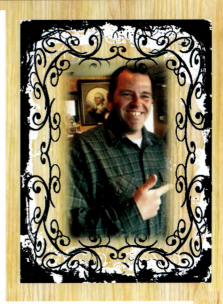

Background: "I was in construction/masonry and a stay-at-home dad. My wife has a master's degree in accounting and worked as a Finance manager at Munson Healthcare. We'd been active for awhile in the local real estate market as landlords. The L.A. Cafe came onto the market and we decided to purchase it and turn it into a brewery. I'd been a home brewer for years and with my skills in construction it seemed like a great match! My wife runs the finance side of things and I brew and schmooze. It works out great!"

What motivates you? "I'm not gonna lie. Money is my big motivator! It's not all I'm out for, obviously, but it is a driving force since we both depend on this place for our livelihood. In order to be successful, we need to have happy customers."

How do you decide what to brew? "At first I went with my gut and what I like. Now, I tend to brew what the customers want."

How do you name your beers? "I lean toward picking a name that amuses me. Like the name *Jungle Fungus*. My mom used to say that our neighbor mowing barefoot had jungle fungus and that's why he didn't like to wear shoes. I also like my names to have a cadence to them."

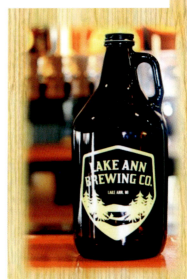

What were your original goals and have they changed? "Our original goal was to be successful in this location since my wife quit her job to enable me to pursue my dream of opening a brewery. Now we really enjoy being self-employed and self-financed. It gives us a great feeling of independence. I can't overstate the relationship our business has with the community, not just our locals here in Lake Ann, but the brewing community as well. We have made many friends and have developed lots of good relationships. It's been very rewarding."

Join us for live Music every night (Tuesday-Saturday) in the summer months.

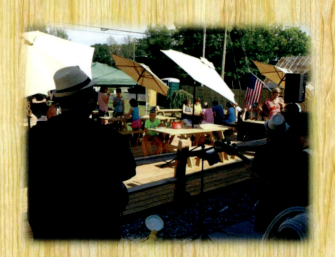
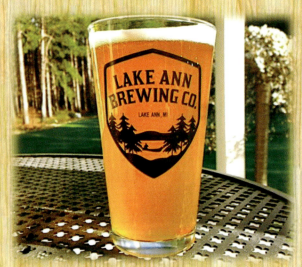
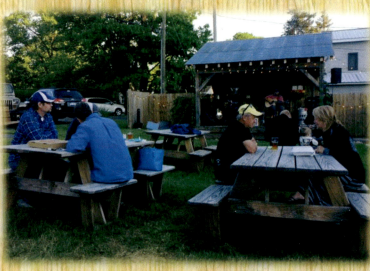
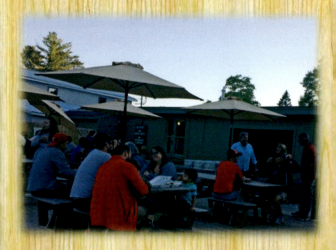

Lake Ann Brewing Co. – Matt Therrien

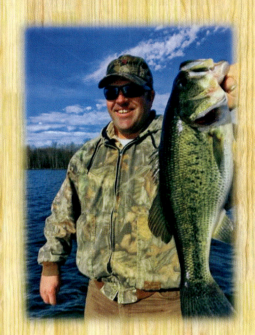

Fun fact: "I don't really enjoy the brewing process, although I have a passion to make great craft beer. Thank goodness I have a great assistant brewer, Nick Hall!"

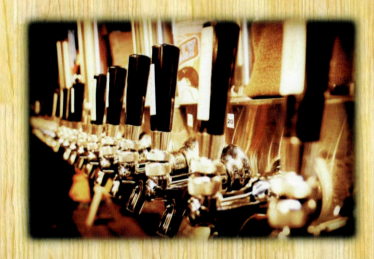

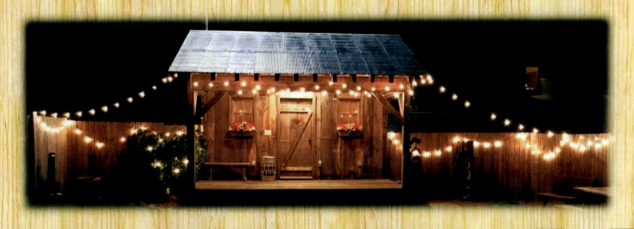

Mackinaw Brewing

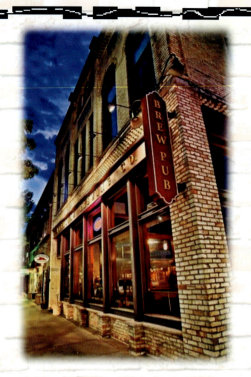

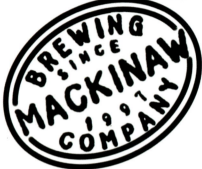

161 East Front Street
Traverse City
mackinawbrewing.com

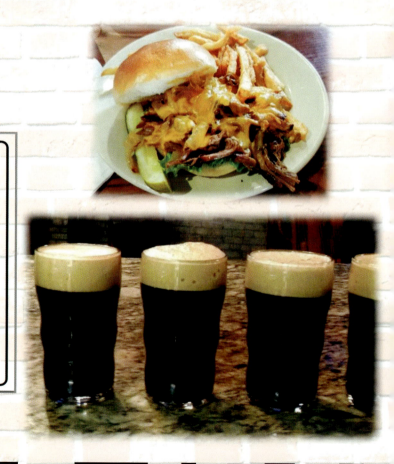

Mackinaw Brewing was the first brewpub to open up in downtown Traverse City.

We specialize in amazing hand-crafted brews, delicious smoked meats, and a fun relaxing atmosphere.

Come on in and engage in some good conversation or just kick back and enjoy a pint.

See ya soon.

Head Brewer: Mike Dwyer

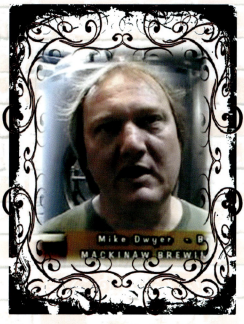

Background: "I was a home brewer for ten years and I wanted to expand my hobby. Mackinaw Brewing was just under construction and I went in to apply for a job and ended up getting the assistant brewer position. The head brewer left after 6 months and **boom** I became the head brewer. Twenty years later – I'm still here."

What **motivates** you? "Brewing beer, making beer. I still really enjoy what I do. It's challenging and it offers stability to my family and I work for good people."

How do you decide **what to brew?** "Often the beer gods strike me out of the blue or I'll be busy doing something and an idea hits me. Other times inspiration comes when I'm drinking a beer or talking to the hop supplier."

How do you **name your beers?** "I'm not very good at beer naming. I tend to lean on the staff and mug club regulars. I tell them what I've brewed and they come up with a list of names for me to choose from."

What were your original goals and have they changed?
"Oh yeah, you bet. I was going to be a musician and I only applied at Mackinaw Brewing to learn more about my hobby. I was planning to go into recording engineering and then things flipped. I make a living brewing and I'm still in a band. I play electric and lap steel guitars in the band we formed for the 10 year anniversary celebration of Mackinaw Brewing Company and we've been playing together ever since."

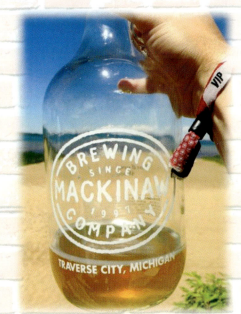

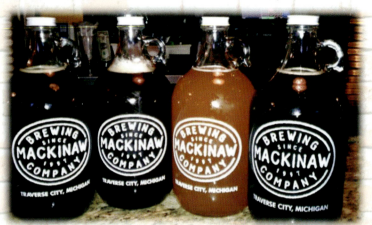

Brew Club:
- Mackinaw Brew Club members meet every Tuesday. Join today to enjoy good company and a lifetime of savings!

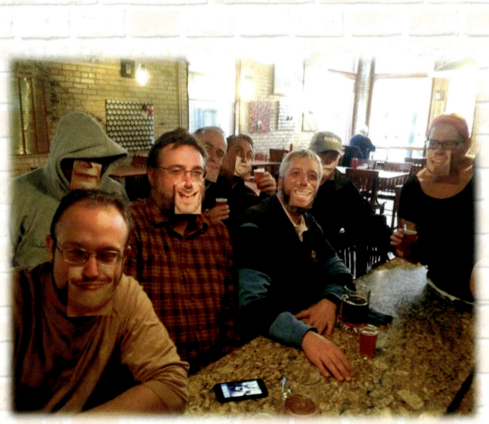

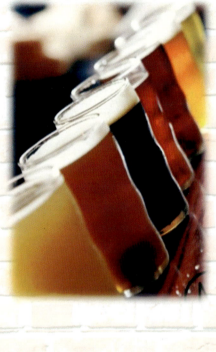

Mackinaw Brewing – Mike Dwyer

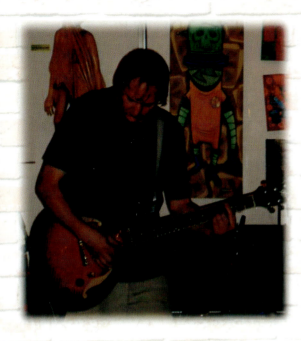

Fun facts:
- Mike plays the electric and lap steel guitars for his three-piece progressive, folk rock band.
- Mike has worked in downtown Traverse City since he was 14 years old.

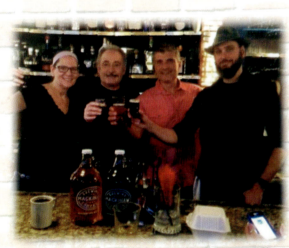

Cheers from our friendly staff!

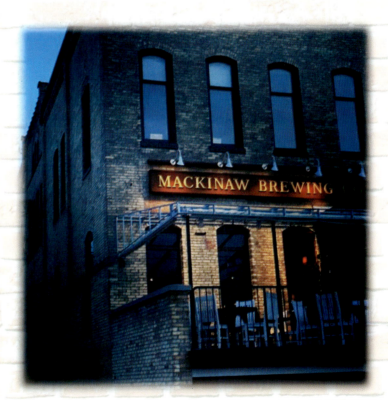

North Peak Brewing Company

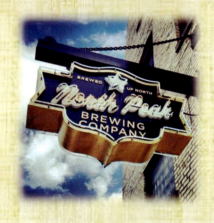

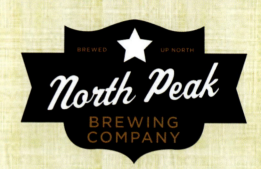

400 West Front Street
Traverse City
northpeak.net

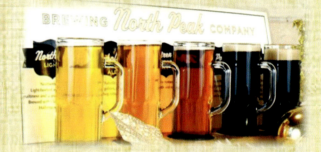

North Peak Brewing Company is located in a historic building which was formerly the Big Daylight Candy Factory. The building is a handsome imposing brick edifice of three floors and a basement. It was constructed with 400,000 bricks and 250,000 feet of lumber, erected and supplied with the latest and most approved machinery devices for the manufacturing of all kinds of candies.

North Peak Services include:
- Lunch, Dinner and Drinks
- Takes Reservations
- Walk-Ins Welcome
- Good For Groups
- Good For Kids
- Take Out
- Waiter Service
- Outdoor Seating

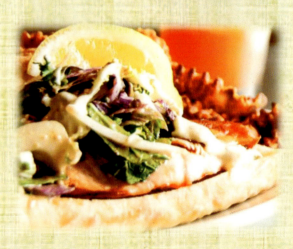

Head Brewer: Dave Hale

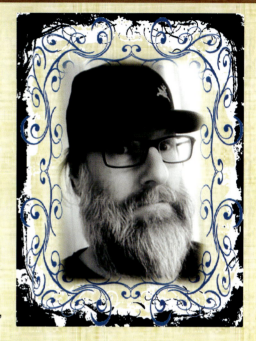

Background: "I began home brewing as a student at Western Michigan University in Kalamazoo, also home to Bell's Brewery. I was fortunate to have a roommate who worked there and also knew the current head brewer, who taught me how to homebrew on a 5 gallon scale. After honing my home brewing skills, I attended the American Brewers Guild in 1996. This led directly to my almost 20 years in the brewing industry. I've been head brewer now at 3 brewpubs and production brewer/cellar man/lab tech at 2 breweries, including Bell's in Kalamazoo and Arcadia Ales in Battle Creek. I'd always wanted to live in Traverse City and also was looking to move out of production brewing back to the brewpub environment. The head brewing position was opening up in May 2010 and I jumped on the opportunity."

What motivates you? "Pride, quality and customer satisfaction are 3 major motivators for me in the workplace. No matter what I'm brewing, my goal is to make the best & most consistent brews possible, following Standard Operating Procedures batch after batch. At the end of the day, I'm happy seeing a bar full of North Peak patrons enjoying the hand-crafted ales we work so hard to produce."

How do you decide what to brew? "With 11 different beers on tap (7 different menu brews + 4 rotating seasonals) the first thing I track is weekly volume depletion of each style. What do I need to brew to keep all these beers on tap? What's going to run out in the next 2-3 weeks? For seasonal brews, I try to offer beers that customers are longing for and are also appropriate for the time of year. I watch for style trends while also gathering inspiration or ideas by sampling beers from other breweries (doesn't matter if it's a local competitor or a brewery from 2,000 miles away). I'm also looking at past specialty brews I've offered. Many I bring back every year, some I don't. If they were popular and/or created a buzz around our pub, I'll brew it again. If it wasn't received with the excitement I'd hoped for or was a slow mover I'll either not try it again or possibly try it in a different season in the future."

How do you name your beers? "Naming beers is sometimes the first thing that intrigues a guest to try a beer, so I do my best to make them interesting and fun, while hopefully conveying some informative aspect regarding the beer. I like to include some local influence as much as possible, but also inject some of my personality and interests. When all else fails I turn to music. Plays on band names, artists and song names is an angle I try to incorporate into my seasonal creations as much as possible."

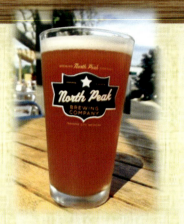

What were your original goals and have they changed? "My original goal or dream was to be an owner/operator of a brewpub or small production brewery. Still dreaming, but I've learned so much in 20 years about business and the industry that I'm ok with the position I'm in. Being head brewer of a brewpub operation has many aspects of ownership. While I don't own anything, I'm responsible for everything we do in the brewery- the equipment, scheduling, raw ingredient inventory, the beers on tap, my assistant's training, development and performance, and finally when's the best time for me to get out of the brewery and recharge."

One More Thing – "Being a professional brewer since 1996, I've seen many changes in the craft industry. Beers and styles (can you say lighter lagers & fruit beers) that were sometimes frowned upon are now being embraced. Being in the middle of the craft brewing boom has been an awesome experience and I'm really happy that I decided to pursue brewing as a career. It's such a rewarding job. It's a labor of love, but at the end of the day it's a great feeling seeing folks enjoying my craft!"

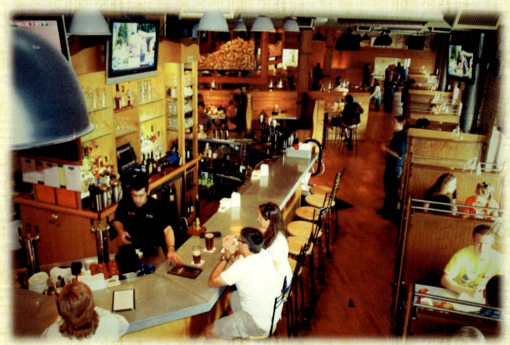

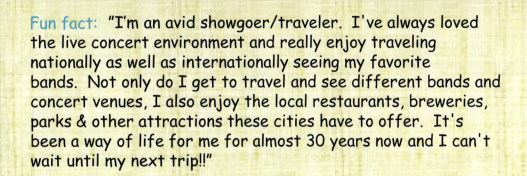

Fun fact: "I'm an avid showgoer/traveler. I've always loved the live concert environment and really enjoy traveling nationally as well as internationally seeing my favorite bands. Not only do I get to travel and see different bands and concert venues, I also enjoy the local restaurants, breweries, parks & other attractions these cities have to offer. It's been a way of life for me for almost 30 years now and I can't wait until my next trip!!"

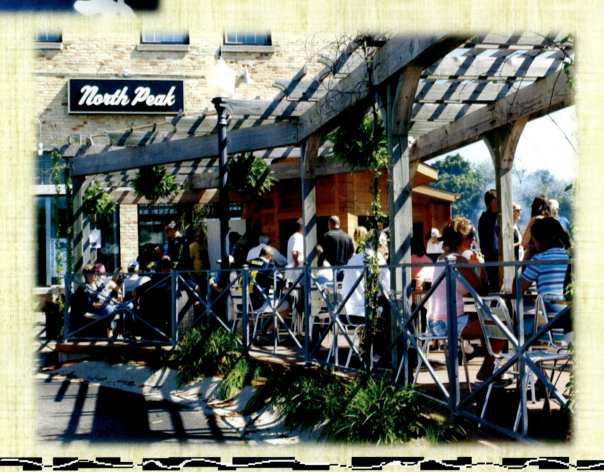

North Peak Brewing Company – Dave Hale

Rare Bird Brewpub

229 Lake Avenue
Traverse City
rarebirdbrewpub.com

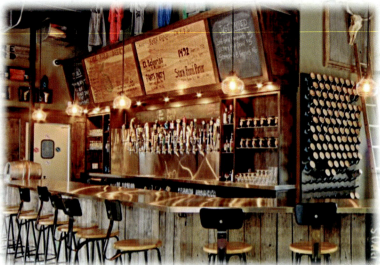
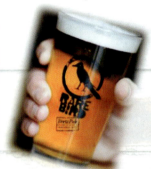
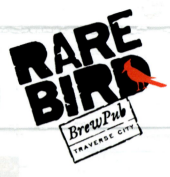
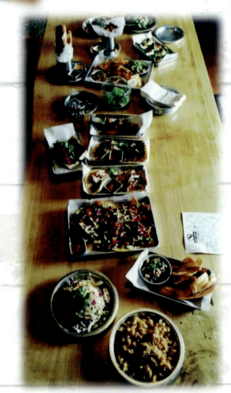

Rare Bird Brewpub is located at 229 Lake Avenue in downtown Traverse City in a beautifully restored, 1931 red brick building. They brew their own beers and also offer a wide range of beers & beverages from other great breweries, wineries & distilleries from Michigan and around the world. The "Bird Food" menu includes starters, salads, sandwiches and entrees including customer favorites like pork belly nachos, kimchi burger and chorizo and potato tacos.

Head Brewer / Co-owner: Tina Schuett

Background: Tina was born and raised in Wisconsin and got interested in beer as a high school exchange student in Germany. She first brewed beer as a college student at Wisconsin-Stevens Point. After working as a park ranger and at a children's health research company she got the idea to try and make a living brewing beer.

What **motivates** you? "I am super competitive even against myself," Tina proudly proclaims. "I always strive to brew better than the last time and I love to beat the local competition in order to prove myself."

How do you decide **what to brew?** "I try to keep an even spread of styles on tap (IPA, pale, light, Belgian and a random selection). Typically, the IPA goes faster and that factors in to brewing schedule to ensure the tanks are always full."

How do you **name your beers?** "I have no set way to name my beer. Sometimes there's a name first that inspires a beer (**Her Name was Amber**). Sometimes the beer is first then the name (**Love Wins**). There are also inside jokes (**Sugar Bits**). I just try to have fun with the naming process." Some of the mainstays include **Pants Party Pale Ale, Still the Dude IPA** and **Large Marge Belgian** special.

What were your original goals and have they changed? "My original goal was simply to make a living brewing beer. I was able to accomplish that goal and 3 years later opened Rare Bird with my business partner Nate Crane. We've been open for 2 ½ years and talk about expanding to other Northern Michigan locations. Even if expansion were to take place, though, I would stick to brewing, a career that I'm still loving."

Local Awards and Recognition

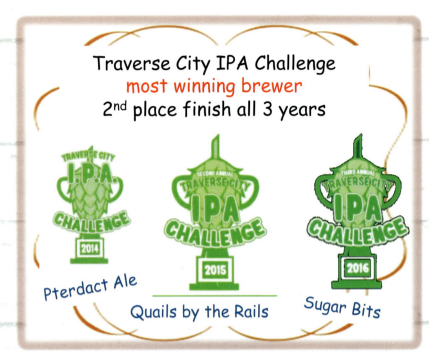

Traverse City IPA Challenge
most winning brewer
2nd place finish all 3 years

Pterdact Ale
Quails by the Rails
Sugar Bits

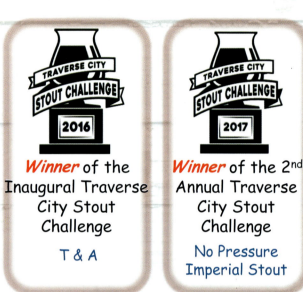

Winner of the Inaugural Traverse City Stout Challenge

T & A

Winner of the 2nd Annual Traverse City Stout Challenge

No Pressure Imperial Stout

Recipient of the 2016 Traverse City Business News **40Under40** given to the region's most influential professionals under the age of 40

MyNorth/Traverse Magazine
Red Hot Best 2016
Northern Michigan Brewers – 3rd place

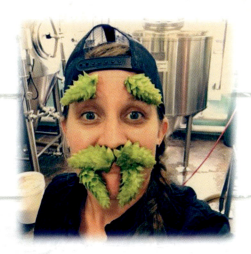

Fun fact: Tina had never brewed an all-grain beer until she landed her first job as a brewer. She'd only brewed extracts.

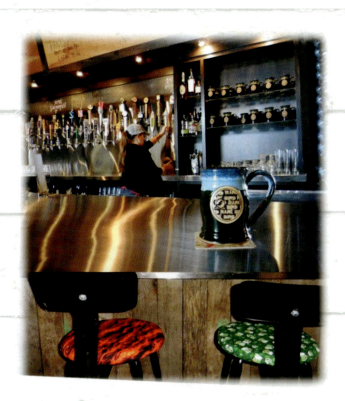

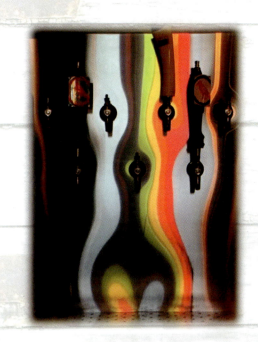

Right Brain Brewery

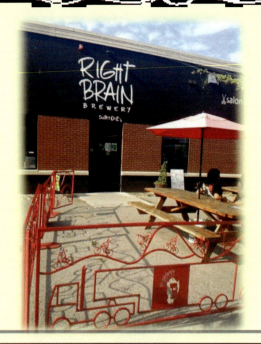

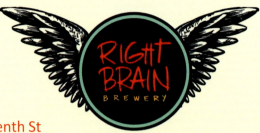

225 East Sixteenth St
Traverse City
rightbrainbrewery.com

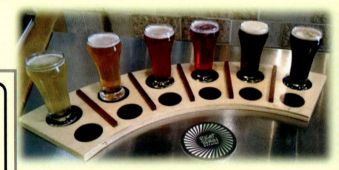

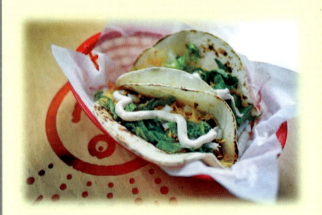

Our stunning new location is a completely renovated and updated warehouse dating back more than 50 years. We've worked hard to reclaim and re-use as much of the old building as possible, while at the same time creating a warm and inviting atmosphere suitable for beer drinking and conversing.

Our beer selection is constantly rotating, and at any time we have between 15 & 25 craft beers on tap. (We only serve our own beer, and that's the way we like it.)

Our food menu features delicious sandwiches and burgers served on fresh, sourdough bread. Or try some fresh house-made guacamole, salsa, fries or tacos.

In addition to serving a selection of locally made wines and ciders, we also have soda pop from Northwoods Soda.

Head Brewer/Owner:
Russell Springsteen

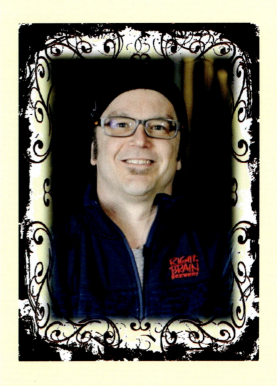

Background: Russ started home brewing in the early 90's in Boulder, Colorado as the craft brew scene was emerging. He became obsessed with brewing and when he moved to Michigan in 1993 he tried unsuccessfully to find a job at one of the few craft breweries in Northern Michigan at that time. Not to be denied, he came up with a business plan and Right Brain was born!

What **motivates** you? "Besides money, I have a fiery passion for good beer. This is a tough business but I love what we do. I love being creative and trying new things. I relish getting people to try beers out of their normal realm."

How do you decide **what to brew?** "I get inspirations. For example, one night I had Pad Thai for dinner and that led to our *Thai Peanut* beer."

How do you **name your beers?** "I try to be creative and make it fun. Often the names are collaborations from our seven brewers. We've used song titles, plays on words and more literal names, like *Dead Kettle*. That name arose because the brew kettle flame kept going out during brewing. Our *Concrete Dinosaur* was named after the brontosaurus shaped concrete mass in the brew room that never got smoothed out after pouring."

What were your original goals and have they changed? "Oh my yes. I originally started out wanting to own a salon with 3 chairs and cut hair. The brewery was to have 8 employees and be a low-key adventure. And then expansion just happened! It was like we were having a backyard bonfire and someone came and poured on gasoline. We now have 37 employees and I only get to cut hair once a month for fun. It's been quite an adventure."

Awards and Recognition

- **GOLD** Medal for **MANGALITSA PIG PORTER**: Great American Beer Festival, Experimental Beer -- 2011
- **SILVER** Medal for **CONCRETE DINOSAUR**: Great American Beer Festival, Rye Beer -- 2015

THE BREWERY
- 2016 Traverse City Ale Trail IPA Challenge Winners -- Dead(er) Kettle
- Can Of The Year Nominee, Brewery Collectibles Club of America, 2014 -- Willpower Pale Ale
- Grand Champion, 2014 Ashley's Brewery Throwdown
- Top 5 Local Breweries In The Nation -- 2013, Answers.Com
- Top 10 Best Breweries in Michigan -- Mlive.com

CEO STOUT
- Michigan's Favorite Stout, 2012 & 2013 -- DrinkMichigan.Org
- Best Stout -- 2013 WGRD Summer Craft Beer Festival
- 90/100 on RateBeer.com

DEAD KETTLE *(IPA)*
- Best IPA -- 2013 WGRD Summer Craft Beer Festival

FAT LAD *(Imperial Russian Stout)*
- Bronze Medal -- 2009 World Beer Expo

FLYING SQUIRREL *(Brown Ale)*
- "13 out of 14" -- Michigan Beer Show Podcast

NAUGHTY GIRL STOUT
- "Top 10" Michigan's Favorite Stout, 2013 -- DrinkMichigan.Org

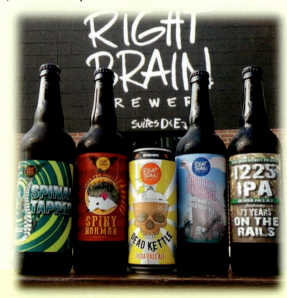

Willpower Pale Ale
- GOLD: World Expo of Beer, Best English Pale Ale, 2015
- 90 out of 100, Draft Magazine, 2014

Smokey CEO Stout
- GOLD: World Expo of Beer, Smoke/Wood Beer -- 2015

SMOOTH OPERATOR
- GOLD: World Expo of Beer, Best Light Hybrid -- 2015
- BEST OF SHOW: World Expo of Beer -- 2015

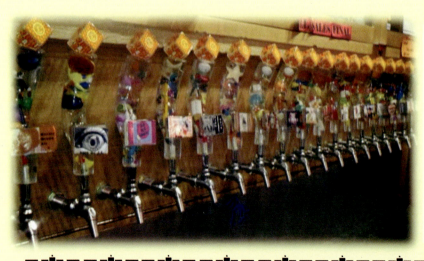

Right Brain Brewery – Russell Springsteen

Fun fact: Russell is a formally trained barber by trade. He cuts and colors both men and women's hair.

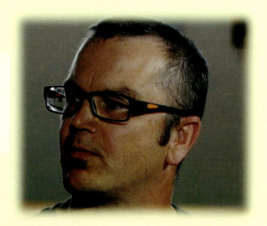

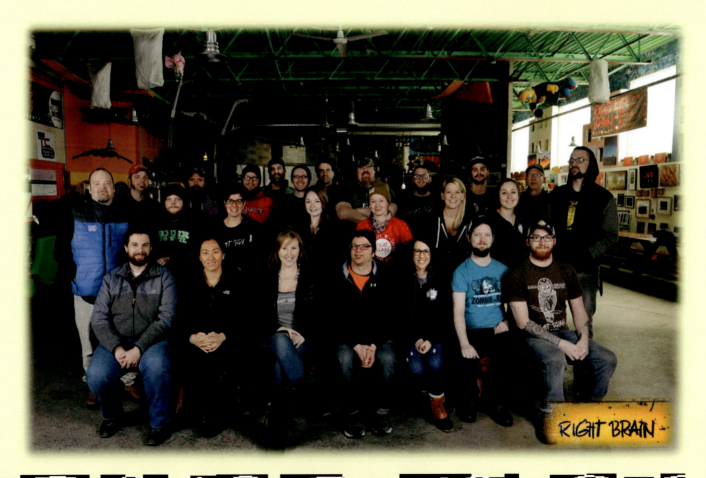

Right Brain Brewery - Russell Springsteen

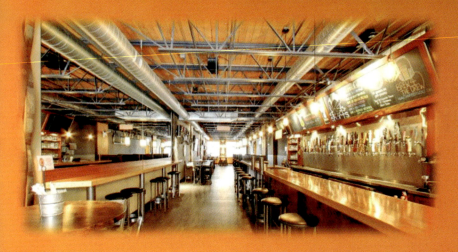

Seven Monks Taproom

128 South Union Street
Traverse City
7monkstap.com

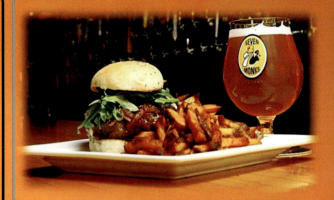

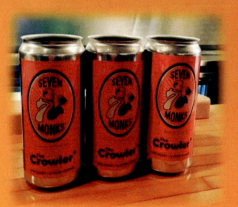

Why the name, 7 Monks Taproom?

Trappist beer are ales brewed by or under control of Trappist monks. Yes, we said monks. There were a total of 174 Trappist monasteries worldwide (as of April 2011); only seven (six in Belgium and one in the Netherlands) produced Trappist beer and were authorized to label their beers with the Authentic Trappist Product logo. Hence the name during 2011 when we first opened.

We love beer. Our beer flows from 46 taps and our ever-changing bottled beer selection. We consistently serve seasonal craft beers from Michigan and around the world.

Come try our food…it's delicious and a lot of it is local! Oh, we also have wine, cider, and local mead on tap.

Certified Cicerone: Jason Kasdorf

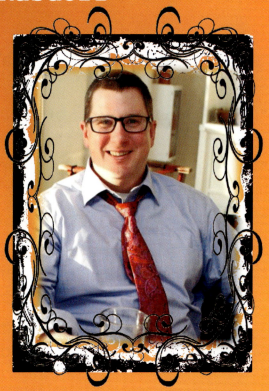

Background: Jason was born in Michigan and moved to Colorado in 1991 just as the craft beer industry was catching on. Although never working in one of the existing breweries there, he was a frequent visitor. When he returned to Michigan in 2011 he applied at the all the local breweries and eventually landed at Seven Monks.

What **motivates** you? "I love the camaraderie and community aspect of my job. The tenacity and competitiveness around me is contagious. My job combines my three favorite things: beer, people and history. What could be better than that?!"

How do you decide what beers to **have on tap?** "I try to keep all the important styles available, including beers from outside the country. I also love to bring in beers based on customer feedback."

What were your original goals and have they changed? "My original goal was simply to get into the beer industry. I like representing all kinds of beer and beer styles. I enjoy the fact that I'm always learning. I'm very interested in the history of beer and I've researched and given talks about the history of brewing in the Traverse City area."

What is the title Cicerone and how do you earn it? Certified Cicerone is the second level of certification. Those who achieve this certification have a solid and well-rounded knowledge of beer and beer service as well as basic competence in assessing beer quality and identity by taste. To earn the title of Certified Cicerone individuals must pass an exam which demonstrates that they possess a professional body of knowledge and essential tasting skills related to beer. This credential has been earned by more than 2,500 people in 19 countries working in nearly every role in the industry from bartenders to brewery presidents.

Awards, Recognition and News

- **DRAFT** Magazine – America's 100 best beer bars, 2016, 2015 and 2014

- THRILLIST – Best 33 Beer Bars in America

- THRILLIST – **Best** Beer Bar in Michigan

- The Awesome Mitten – Best 14 Beer Bars in Michigan

- Come visit us at our brother locations!
    Seven Monks has two additional locations:
    - Boyne City (opened in July 2016)
    - Grand Rapids (opened in April 2017)

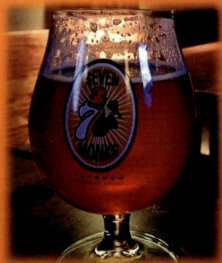

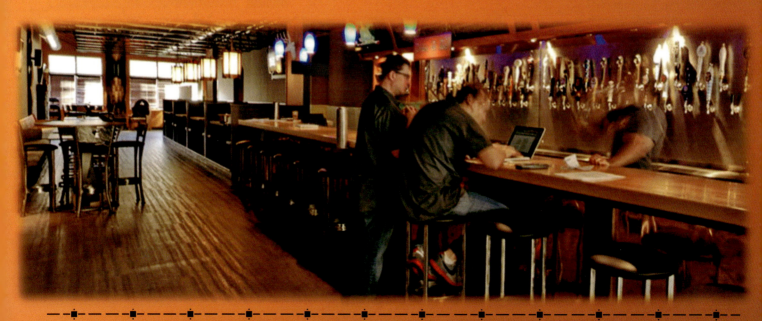

Seven Monks Taproom – Jason Kasdorf

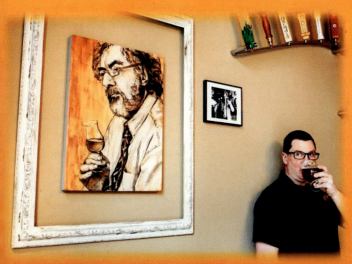

Fun fact: Before getting into the beer business, Jason designed and manufactured brass and copper wire sculptures.

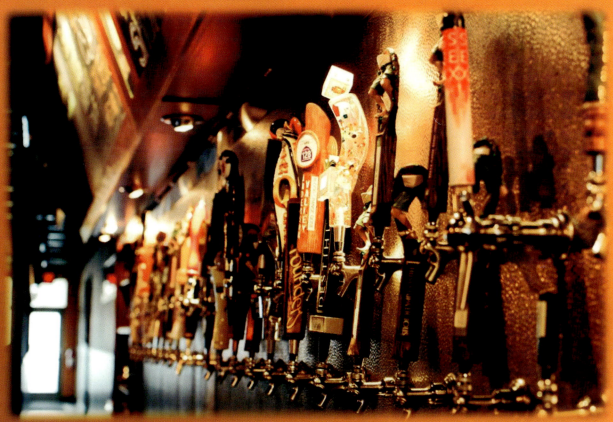

Short's Brewing Company

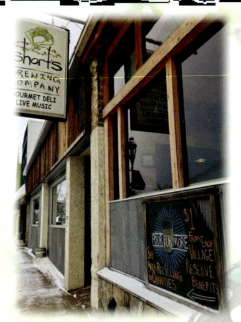

121 N. Bridge Street, Bellaire and
211 Industrial Park Drive, Elk Rapids
shortsbrewing.com

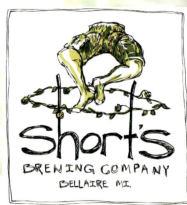

Short's Manifesto!

WE EXIST
to enrich the lives of people around us and for the betterment of planet earth.

WE TAKE PRIDE
in crafting high quality, creatively fearless beer.
in fostering ambition and imagination.
in building consumer appreciation by spreading excitement for our craft through Beer Liberation.

WE STRIVE
to be Michigan's craft brewery.

WE LOVE
what we do and where we live.

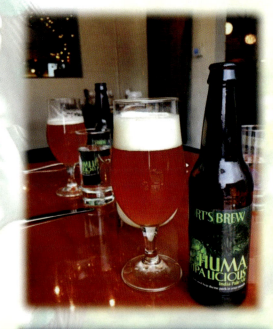

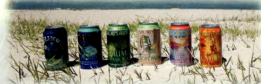

Short's Brewing Head Brewer:
Tony Hansen

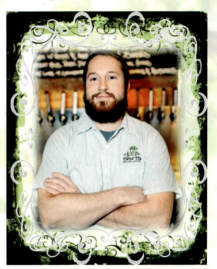

Background: "I grew up in Buckley, MI and graduated from Buckley Community Schools. I began cooking at Boone's Long Lake Inn at the age of 16 and continued cooking while attending Northwestern Michigan College. I also dabbled in organic farming, biofuel production, converting cars to run on vegetable oil, winemaking, cidermaking and homebrewing. Homebrewing became my favorite hobby, and I decided to research brewing as a profession. I met Joe Short in late 2006 while seeking advice from brewers on how to get started in the industry. Joe mentioned that he needed help at Short's and I quickly accepted a job at Short's as a part-time brewer. The part-time brewer position rapidly changed to full-time brewer within the first year. I am now the Head Brewer at Short's."

What **motivates** you? "Originally, I was motivated to make beer that people would not only enjoy drinking, but really find unique and entertaining. I was motivated to create an experience to share, talk about, and remember. I tried to create intensely flavored beer, but also give it fun and interesting names and images. After witnessing many positive reactions to that approach, I decided to continue on the same path. The creativity allowed in brewing Short's brews continues to motivate me."

How do you decide **what to brew?** "I have a huge list of beer ideas that I work from. Most of my decisions are based off of what type of beer would work seasonally and round out our current offerings. But really, whatever sounds like the most fun and interesting idea normally makes it to the top of the list. I also like to bring back a lot of previously brewed beers based off of demand."

How do you **name your beers?** "I have a few methods for naming beers. The first is the most straightforward and obvious which is to call the beer exactly what it's intended to taste like. For example, if the concept is to make a beer taste like key lime pie, I'll call it **Key Lime Pie**. The other common method is more like a game of beer association. The beer is associated with some sort of an idea or inside joke that is happening around the time the beer is conceived or brewed and that's what we base the name on. The final method requires a little magical brewer thinking. I form a character that reflects the ingredients or style of the beer which leads to a name that fits that character."

What were your original goals and have they changed? "My original goal was to be a pub brewer with unlimited creative freedom, which I attained at Short's. But as Short's has grown and my position at the brewery has changed and as I've become a father and family man, my goals have changed. My goals are now centered around doing whatever I can to contribute to Short's continued success in order to support my coworkers and their families, as well as mine."

Awards and Recognition

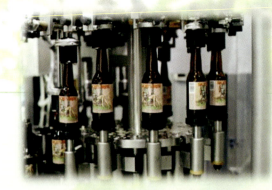

THE BREWERY: 2010 RateBeer.com Best Beers in the World
- #64 – 100 Best Brewers in the World
- #5 – 50 Best Brewpubs

THE BEER
- **SILVER** Medal for **MELT MY BRAIN**: Great American Beer Festival, Experimental Beer - 2015
- **GOLD** Medal for **KEY LIME PIE**: Great American Beer Festival, Experimental Beer – 2014
- Draft Magazine Top 25 Beers of the Year for **THE GAMBLER** – 2011
- **GOLD** Medal for **KEY LIME PIE**: Great American Beer Festival, Experimental Beer – 2010
- **BRONZE** Medal for **BLACK LICORICE LAGER**: World Beer Cup, Herb & Spice Beer /Chocolate Beer – 2010
- **SILVER** Medal for **BLOODY BEER**: Great American Beer Festival, Experimental Beer - 2009

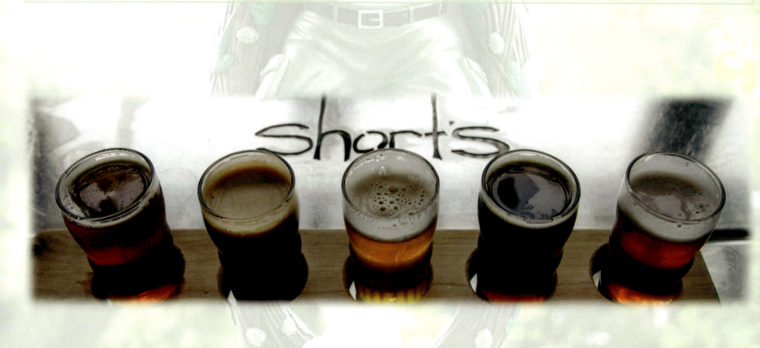

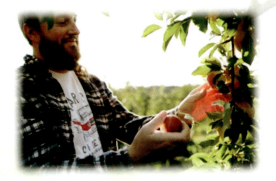

Fun fact: "I lived on site at the production facility during the first year of operation."

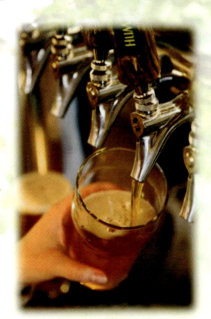

CEO / Creative Engineer: Joe Short

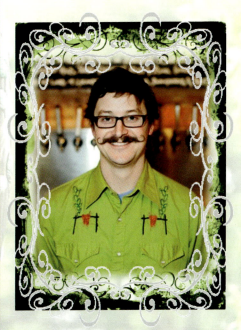

Joe grew up in Rapid City and graduated from Kalkaska High School. He began working in the hospitality industry at a young age as a waiter at the Dockside on Torch Lake. Joe began homebrewing while attending Western Michigan University. After beginning his professional brewing career with stints at the former Traverse Brewing Company in Elk Rapids, the former Michigan Brewing Company in Webberville and the former Jackson Brewing Company (later Zig's Kettle and Brew), Joe decided to return to northern Michigan and start his own brewery. Since then, Joe has worked every position at Short's. Don't be surprised if you stop by our pub and find him pouring beers and taking orders. Behind the scenes, however, Joe spearheads the creative process, any construction or expansion projects, marketing, special events and overall direction of the company. Joe is married to Leah Short, and they have two sons.

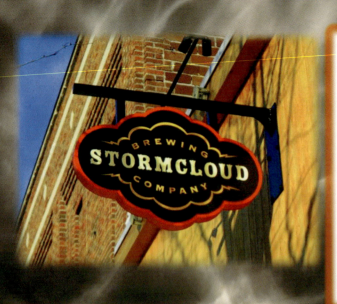

Stormcloud Brewing

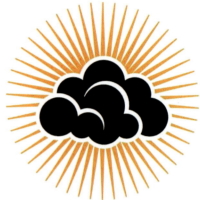

303 Main Street
Frankfort
stormcloudbrewing.com

Belgian-inspired, Michigan-made beer and locally inspired food. Brewery and pub two blocks from lake Michigan in downtown Frankfort.

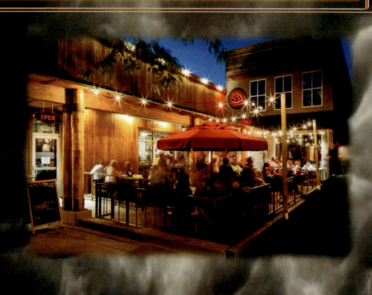

Head Brewer / Co-Owner: Brian Confer

Background: "I worked as a commercial photographer in the area, starting with a stint at *Traverse Magazine* before going freelance. Retirement prospects for a photographer in such a small market are difficult so I started looking at alternative careers. One of my photoshoots for Traverse was with Joe Short at Short's Brewing. I love the combo of food and beer and I thought Short's got it right and I started brainstorming how I could start my own brewery. I drew up my business plan and started home brewing. As luck would have it, I was chatting with friends and acquaintances about my idea and Rick Schmitt was intrigued. We began to talk more seriously and here we are. We have a great partnership. Our skills mesh really well. Rick brings his expertise in the finance and business side, having worked at Crystal Mountain as VP in sales and marketing, and I bring the brewing and creativity.

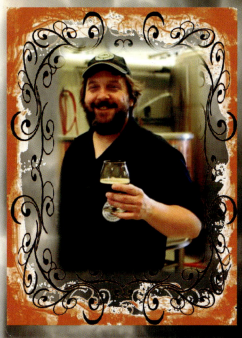

What motivates you? "I moved to Northern Michigan with a degree in fine art and that drive to create is still at the root of everything I do. Rick and I strive to create a cohesive work of art. It's exciting to keep creating, not just beer, but the whole experience."

How do you decide what to brew? "Our base menu is well established and we typically bring in seasonals to fill the cracks. I am partial to Saisons and like to bring fruit into them. I keep a running collection of ideas that I jot down as they come to me and when I need a new beer I hit that idea bank. In the winter we have been brewing a dark and stormy film series that's been a lot of fun. We brew a dark strong to pair with our movie features (3 each winter). For example, this past winter we brewed *Ea and the Goddess* to go with the movie *The Brand New Testament*. The beer was named for Ea, one of the main characters, and featured ingredients from the Last Supper (figs, dates, nutmeg, cinnamon and pistachios)."

How do you name your beers? "I like to make them like book titles – a two or three word phrase that refers to an underlying story or personality, like *The Farthest Shore* or The *Nightswimmer*. I also like wordplay with literary references like *B., Sirius*. Names are a part of the identity of the beer. I may brew a batch a bit differently but I keep the name."

What were your original goals and have they changed? "I started out just wanting to be successful outside photography. Our goal now is to keep moving forward with current growth and use it to meet more people, live an engaging and thoughtful life, and play a positive role in the community. We want to keep our sense of adventure and see how far we can take it."

Awards and Recognition

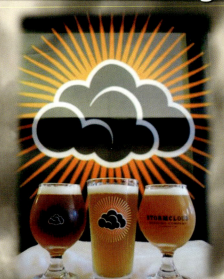

Named one of "Michigan's 50 Companies to Watch" in 2016 by the Michigan Celebrates Small Business Association

Winner of the 2014 Great American Beer Festival *Bronze Medal* in the Belgian Style-Blonde Ale or Pale Ale category

Rainmaker

MyNorth/Traverse Magazine
Red Hot Best 2016
Northern Michigan Brewers – 2nd place

Winner of the 2016 Mlive – Best New Brewery in Michigan

Named in May 2017 as one of "Lower Michigan's Five Breweries to Visit" by Hour Detroit

Stormcloud Brewing – Brian Confer

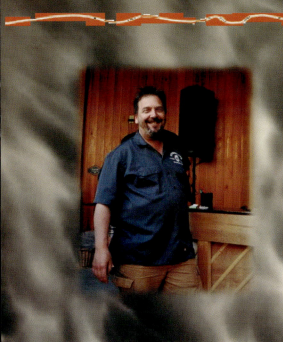

Fun fact: "For every beer at Stormcloud, I create a playlist that plays while the beer is being brewed. This is normally popular with the staff, the exception being the Christmas beer playlists in October!"

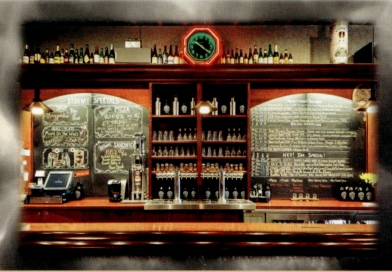

Bulldozers and backhoes broke ground in January 2017 at the future site of Stormcloud's beer production facility.

Located on the east side of the city of Frankfort, the 12,700-square-foot facility will house a 20-barrel brewhouse with the capacity to brew 4,500 barrels of beer per year. Currently, Stormcloud's downtown Frankfort brewery has the capacity to brew 1,200 barrels annually.

The new facility will provide space to install an automated canning line for the purpose of canning a select handful of our best-selling brews for distribution. We also plan to hand-bottle a selection of our traditional Belgian ales in small quantities.

The facility will also include a public tasting room and retail outlet, but those components will NOT open for the 2017 summer. When construction is complete, our primary focus is to brew more beer. Production at the new facility is scheduled to begin summer 2017.

Stormcloud Brewing – Brian Confer

The Filling Station Microbrewery

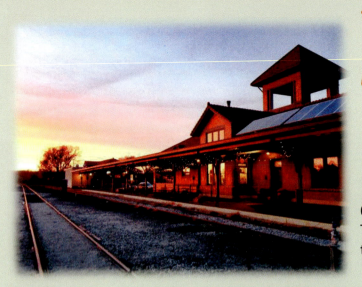

642 Railroad Place
Traverse City
thefillingstationmicrobrewery.com

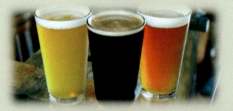

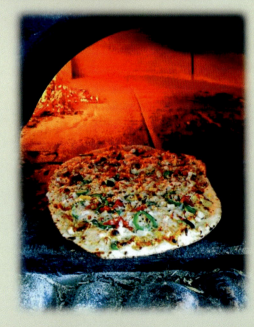

Established in the spring of 2012, The Filling Station Microbrewery is a family owned and operated business, dedicated to providing friendly and knowledgeable service and the highest quality of hand crafted brews and edibles. Located just off the TART Trail in the historic railroad district, the Filling Station Microbrewery features a rotating list of at least 10 craft beers, which pair perfectly with our wood-fired flatbreads and fresh salads. Whether on your own, meeting friends or with your family, patrons of all ages feel welcomed in our casual pub-style setting. You'll enjoy views of Boardman Lake from inside the pub or out on the patio, live music and the occasional train passing by. So whether traveling by car, on foot, riding your bike down the Tart Trail, or paddling across the lake, we invite you to stop by and become a part of the Filling Station family.

The Filling Station Microbrewery – Andy Largent

Head Brewer: Andy Largent

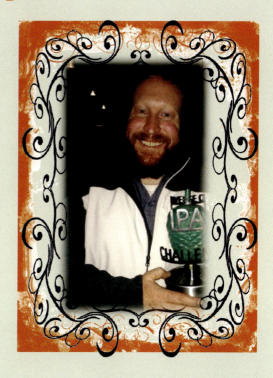

Background: Andy started as a home brewer with mixed results so he wanted to figure out how to brew better beer. At age 21, he was attending NMC, planning to transfer to Ferris State when he landed a job at North Peak with Kim Schneider. He enjoyed it so much he cancelled transferring plans and stuck with brewing. He worked at Right Brain, Stormcloud and Grand Traverse Distillery before landing the head brewing job at the Filling Station Microbrewery.

What **motivates** you? "I like to keep progressing and creating beer everyone enjoys! I enjoy new experiences and learning new brewing techniques."

How do you decide **what to brew?** "I check our brew board and balance recipes so we don't have too much of one style. I consult with the staff and owners for unique ideas, chat with other brewers and read forums, journals and blogs for the latest trends."

How do you **name your beers?** "Beer naming is usually left to Todd (one of the owner's) based on the train theme; like train stops, train lines or geographical locations. For example, **Hop Line IPA**, **Port Huron Pale Ale** and **Union Brown Ale**"

What were your original goals and have they changed? "My original goal was to own a brewery or be a head brewer. I've achieved my head brewer goal and I'm still enjoying it. I like to keep honing recipes. I'm excited about the future of craft brewing in Northern Michigan and I'm happy to be part of it!"

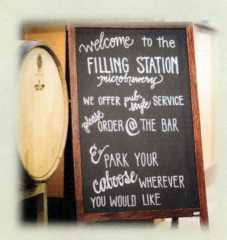

The Filling Station Microbrewery – Andy Largent

About The Depot

In July of 1880, passenger trains arrived in Traverse for the first time via the Chicago and West Michigan Railroad. While these first trains were met by an excited crowd of onlookers, the first permanent freight and passenger depots were not completed until the fall of 1890. The original passenger depot was located east of Union Street, right next to the Hannah Lay grist mill. The freight depot still stands today at the corner of Cass and Lake. The next significant change came in 1899 when the C&WM combined with the Flint & Pere Marquette and the Detroit, Grand Rapids and Western to form the Pere Marquette Railroad. For the next few decades, the use of these rails continued to grow.

Awards and Recognition

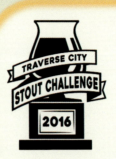
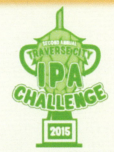
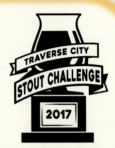

3rd place - Inaugural Traverse City Stout Challenge
Deep Water Imperial Stout

Winner of the 2nd Annual Traverse City IPA Challenge
Wobbly double IPA

2nd place - 2nd Annual Traverse City Stout Challenge
Jacktown Imperial Stout

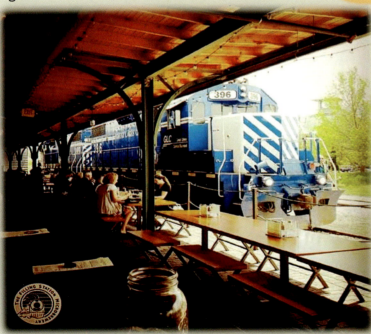

With business booming, the Pere Marquette made the decision to build a new Traverse City Depot on Boardman Lake.
On January 6, 1927, the brand new depot opened to high acclaim, with railroad officials claiming it as the finest station along the entire Pere Marquette line. It has certainly stood the test of time, as this depot continues to thrive as the current home of the Filling Station Microbrewery!

Credit for the information in this brief history:
– "Sail & Rail: A Narrative History of Transportation in the Traverse City Region", by Lawrence & Lucille Wakefield.

The Filling Station Microbrewery – Andy Largent

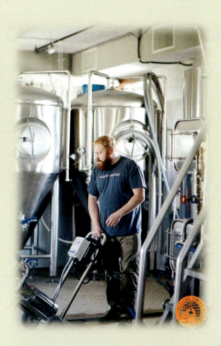

Fun fact: Back in the day, Andy worked as a hot air balloon pilot and crew member for Grand Traverse Balloons.

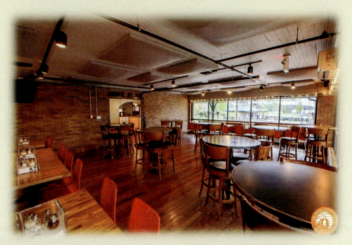

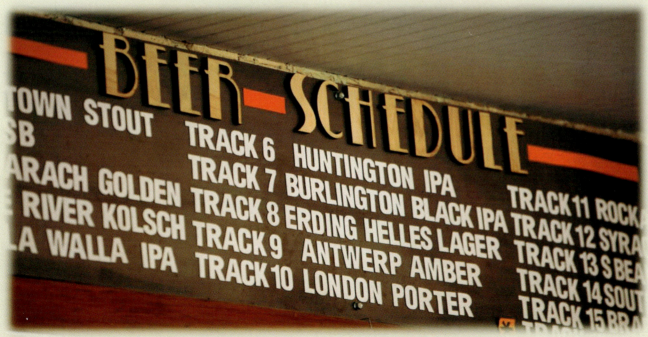

The Mitten Brewing Co.

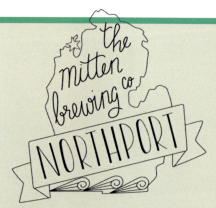

112 W. Nagonaba Street
Northport
mittenbrewing.com

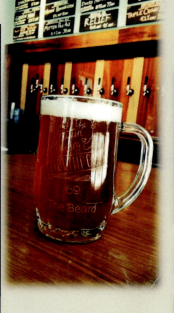

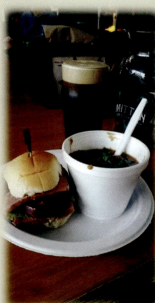

Nestled in the center of historic Northport, Mitten Northport offers guests a chance to enjoy their favorite Mitten tap selections while taking in the view of Grand Traverse Bay and Northport Marina. The taproom, located on the main street of the cozy town, provides an intimate setting for both local and visiting guests.

The taproom proudly offers unique examples of classic beer with 14 styles on tap, as well as wine and cider from local producers. On-site eats are available in the taproom (light fare) or from partnering local food trucks.

With a welcoming bar setting, a covered outdoor patio featuring a ginormous stone fireplace, and backyard bier garden, Mitten Northport is the perfect place to enjoy craft beer in the most picturesque village in Leelanau County.

Taproom Manager: Dan Frank

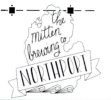

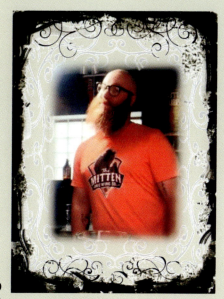

Background: "I was born and raised in Northport. In 2014 when Northport Brewing opened I started hanging out there. Soon after, I was hired as taproom manager which is still my title at The Mitten. When Northport Brewing closed in 2016 The Mitten from Grand Rapids took over. We currently don't have a brewer on site. We serve beers from The Mitten Grand Rapids location. However, we recently received our license to begin brewing again and our plan is to have a brewer on-site and brewing soon. We will focus on sour and barrel aged beers and maybe some test batches unique to our Northport location."

What motivates you? "It's a great industry and it's a lot of fun. It's hard not to enjoy it. In my previous career, I was a mechanic. I now joke that at least people are now happy to see me!"

How do you decide what to brew? "We do have some input into what beers we have on tap. Besides our flagship beers and award winners, we also try to keep up with what's moving in our taproom."

How do you name your beers? "The Mitten in Grand Rapids is a vintage baseball-themed microbrewery/pizzeria. So beer names play off that theme. For example, **Docks No-No DIPA** was named after Dock Ellis's no hitter that he pitched while under the influence of LSD."

What were your original goals and have they changed? "My original goals were to make the taproom inviting for both tourists and locals. I think we've done a good job of that. Even with the addition of brewing, I think our goals will remain the same, but we'll be a legit brewery, not just a bar serving craft beers."

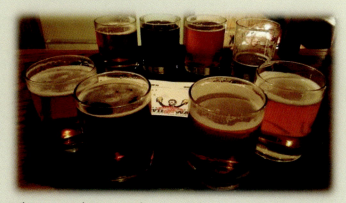

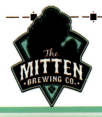

Awards and Recognition

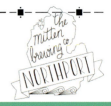

Featured on Food Network's *Burgers, Brew & 'Que* (Northport location)

Winner of the 2017 World Expo of Beer *Gold Medal* in the Brown British beer style category

Triple Crown Brown Ale

Winner of the 2017 World Expo of Beer *Silver Medal* in the American IPA beer style category

Country Strong IPA

In 2015, received the "President's Award" from the Association of Fundraising Professionals for the company's charitable giving program, the Mitten Foundation.

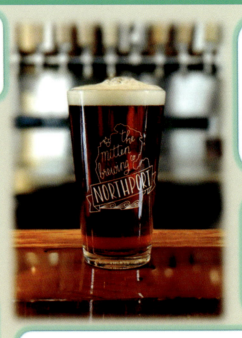

Winner of the 2013 Mlive – Michigan's Best New Brewery (Grand Rapids location)

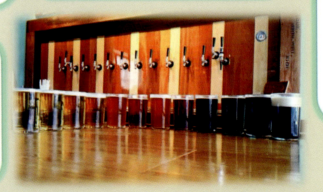

Winner of the 2016 Great World Beer Cup *Silver Medal* in the English Style Mild Ale beer style category

Triple Crown Brown Ale

Finalist for "2014 Beverage Newsmaker of the Year" in the Grand Rapids Business Journal (Grand Rapids location)

Recognized in 2015 as "Young Entrepreneurs of the Year" by the Grand Rapids Chamber of Commerce

The Mitten Brewing Co. – Dan Frank

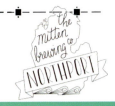

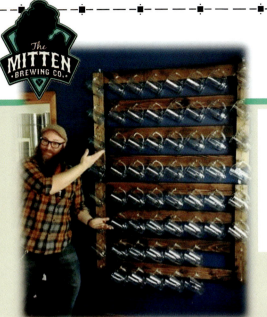

Fun fact: "My mom's family dates back to when the village of Northport was settled and missionaries warned the local Indians that 'the white man is coming'."

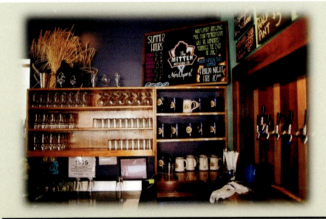

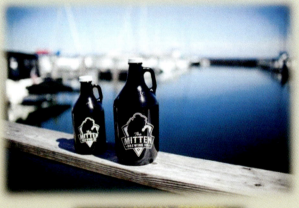

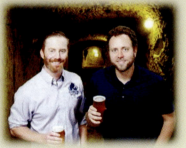

Co-owners, Chris Andrus and Max Trierweiler

The Mitten Brewing Company was founded in November 2012 by lifelong friends Chris Andrus and Max Trierweiler. With locations in Grand Rapids and Northport, The Mitten is a vintage baseball-themed Michigan microbrewery with a focus on community involvement and charitable giving. Andrus and Trierweiler were dedicated homebrewers who saw an opportunity to broaden the state's craft beer scene and also have an impact on the community at large.

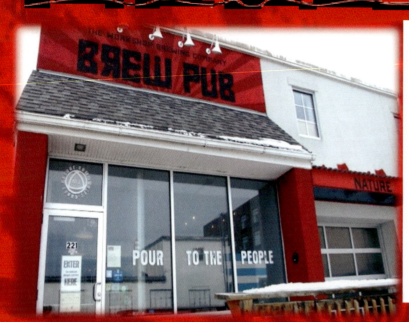

The Workshop Brewing Company

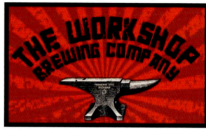

221 Garland Street
Traverse City
traversecityworkshop.com

The Workshop Brewing Company exists to preserve Northern Michigan's spectacular natural environment, to reinforce Traverse City's warm and vital community, and to honor traditional craft. We do not consider our business to be a success unless we are demonstrably and sustainably doing all three. We express this commitment by using the Trifidelity symbol, which stands for our motto: **Nature. Community. Craft.**

Our menu emphasizes fresh, seasonal ingredients, and showcases the incomparable products of local farmers, bakers, and other artisans. It is curated to be the perfect complement to our Heirloom Beers. Various snacks, salads, soups, and specials round out the menu.

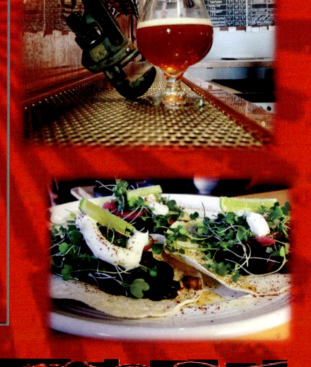

The Workshop Brewing Company – Michael Wooster

Head Brewer: Michael Wooster

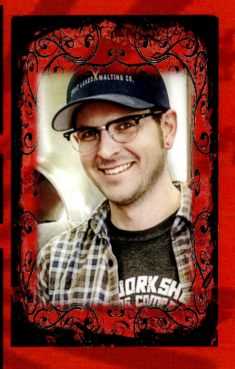

Background: Michael started out working part time in a winery while working as a full-time cook in a local restaurant. He liked the winery environment, but not the wine. He was home brewing at that time and decided he wanted to explore working in a brewery. He helped out at local breweries until he eventually landed a full time brewing position.

What motivates you? "My family motivates me and knowing that I can support them doing something that I'm enthusiastic about gives me satisfaction."

How do you decide what to brew? "We have some set menu beers that are pub favorites and we have a series of seasonals. Additional beers might be just a style we want to try or some special brew that I want to make myself. We are currently working on a collaboration with local adventure tour Kayak, Bike and Brew to provide a lighter lager brewed with lemon peel."

How do you name your beers? "We try to name our beers to go along with the theme of the workshop. Most of the names are names of tools. A one-off brew may have a non-tool name, but anything that will stick around is named after a tool. For example, **Ten-Pound Sledge IPA, Ball Peen ESB** and **Sickle Saison**."

What were your original goals and have they changed? "I've always had a dream to own my own brewery. That hasn't happened yet, but who knows what the future may bring! For now, I am happy to get to work in a career that I enjoy so much."

The Workshop Brewing Company - Michael Wooster

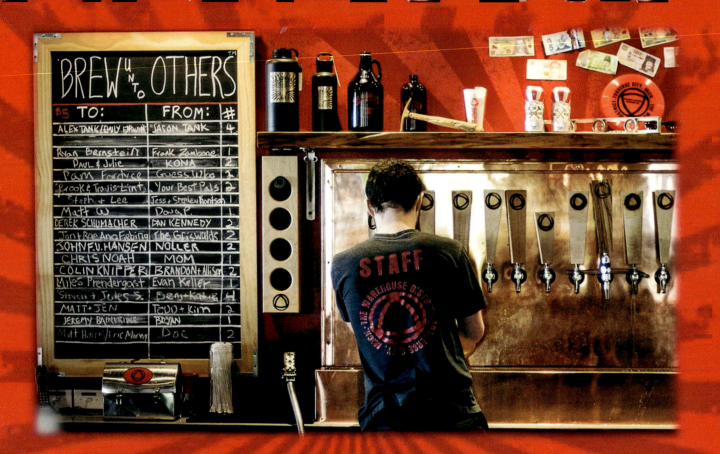
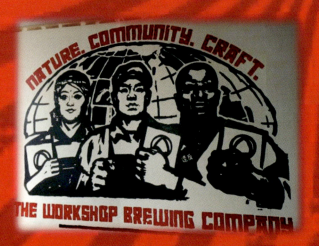
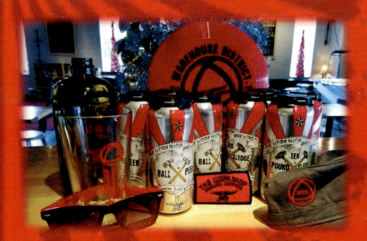

The Workshop Brewing Company – Michael Wooster

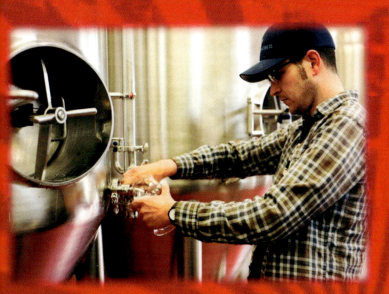

Fun fact: As a high school student, at Traverse City West, Michael was the vocalist in a metal band that toured around the state.

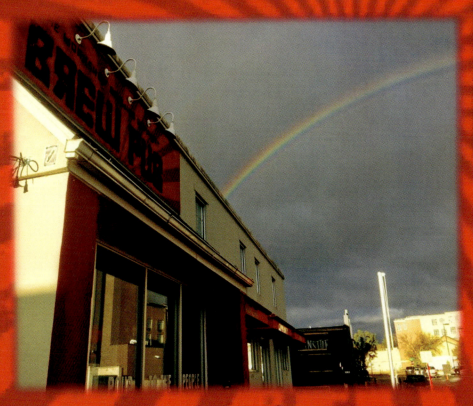

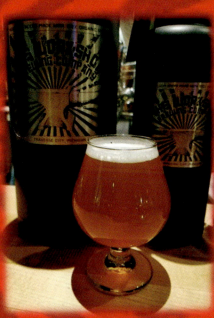

The Workshop Brewing Company - Michael Wooster

Fresh Roots Organic Growers

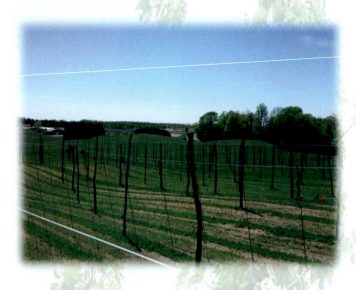

6252 E Harrys Road
Traverse City
joeldmulder.wixsite.com

F.R.O.G. is the first commercial hopyard built 100% organic in Michigan. No synthetic chemicals in our ground, trellis or products from the start in 2009. We specialize in boutique hops and have 14 different varieties, some you can't find anywhere else. We are taking the next step and adding unique organic adjuncts for brewers to our production line. Stay tuned...

F.R.O.G is now home to Crooked Barn Brewing LLC as well. Making custom beverages with products from the farm and surrounding area. Look for it on tap in Traverse City.

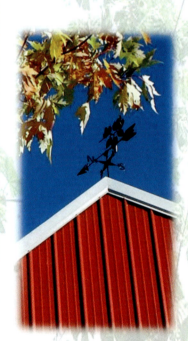

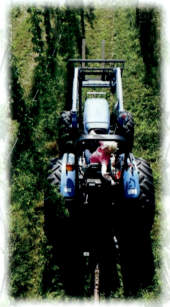

Founder / Owner: Joel Mulder

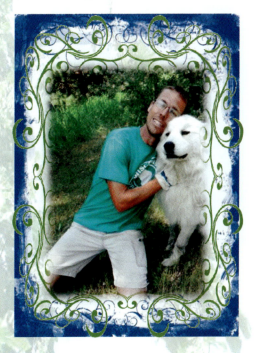

Background: "My educational background is in botany and ecology. Ten years ago I was teaching high school in Cleveland when my wife and I decided to follow my wife's job and move to Traverse City. I couldn't find a teaching job so I decided to try farming. We bought land in Leelanau County and started an organic farm. I was a home brewer so I was interested in hops. Hops are amazing from a botanist point of view. Since I'm a first generation farmer there was lots to learn. Being one who prefers the non-conventional path, I choose to grow organic and to be sustainable. I often implement what some may consider strange ideas, like using sheep for weed control. I got that idea from a Michigan State-sponsored program that included a trip to New Zealand. I came home and bought a couple old ewes on Craigslist."

What **motivates** you? "Being a teacher, I love to educate. I really enjoy showing others my methods. Since I didn't learn farming from my Dad I had so much to learn, but on the flip side, I was not stuck in old ideas and ways of doing things. I love opening people to new ideas and being part of a new crop. Sometimes I even get phone calls from strangers around the state calling with growing questions. I like to call myself 'the underground hop consultant'."

How do you decide **what to grow?** "I talk to brewers, basically. I stay super local. I currently am working with Mackinaw Brewing, The Filling Station, Brewery Terra Firma and Monkey Fist."

What is your **toughest challenge?** "My biggest challenge I have on the farm is balancing cost and need of labor. I'm too small to attract workers or even keep them on for any appreciable time, however, large enough that I can't do it all on my own."

What were your original goals and have they changed? "My original goals were to provide a local, more sustainable product for the local craft brewing scene. I wanted to grow and grow. But, as I got going I found that what I'm really in tune with is the relationships with the brewers. And so my focus is now on those one-on-one relationships."

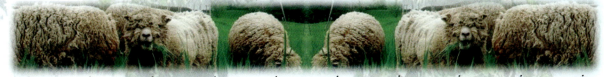

Fresh Roots Organic Growers

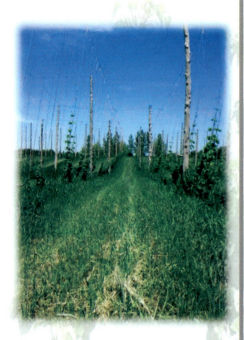

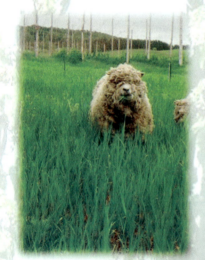

In 2009 Fresh Roots built the first 100% organic commercial hop trellis in Michigan. We chose to be organic not because of the growing trend in the organic market, not because it makes a healthier beer (let's be honest, if you are drinking enough beer that the pesticides contributed by the hops are an issue, you've got bigger problems), but because we believe it's the right way to farm. Nature is put together in certain cycles and mechanisms that keep it running smoothly. Conventional farming has moved too far away from these. At F.R.O.G. farms we try our best to follow these rules and the label "organic" best fits the way we do it.

It definitely wasn't the easy way. The nearest source we could find of untreated 22' poles that would survive the elements were red cedar harvested out of New Jersey. Hops were just starting to return to the area with only a few small experimental yards planted at that time. Brewers were interested in locally produced hops, but also very leery of it. It was a scary time to start out in the hop world.

Since that time, Michigan has since become 4th in production of hops in the United States, and brewers are clamoring for local grown hops. Both sets of our parents have put in countless hours of work and childcare to get the farm going. My wonderful sister joined us in the farm venture to make it even more of a family farm and allowed us to add infrastructure, varieties and a small flock of sheep to help with the weeding. It wasn't always easy, but we're glad we stuck it out.

Fresh Roots now has 13 varieties of hops in production with more on the way. We are proud to serve the area breweries with fresh, local, organic products. We are now looking into expanding our production into brewing adjuncts and spices. Hops are the main crop here at F.R.O.G. farms, but diversity is the spice of life and also is required to put together those natural mechanisms. We also do some vegetables for sale to local farmers markets, as well as fruit, eggs and sheep.

With all of this working together as well as the hard work of the wonderful community of family and friends we have helping us along the way, we are *growing nature's best flavors, the way nature intends.*

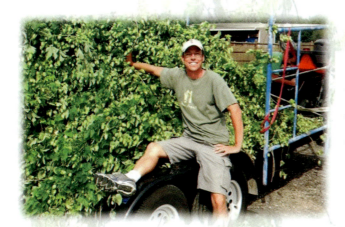

Fun fact: Joel is a stay-at-home dad for his two beautiful children, nine year old daughter, Adeline, and six year old son, Eliott.

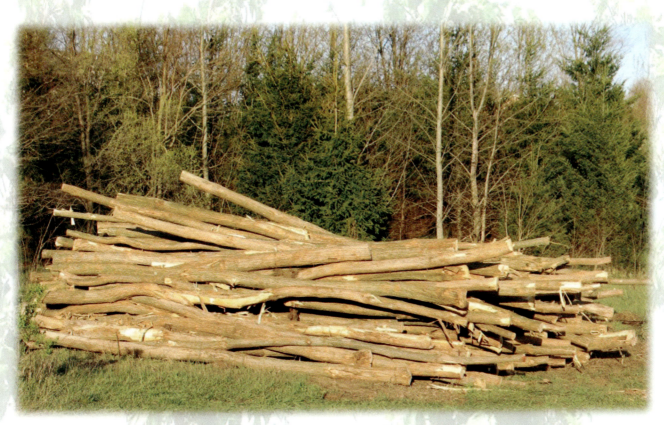

Fresh Roots Organic Growers – Joel Mulder

Great Lakes Malting Co.

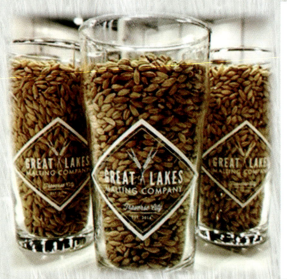

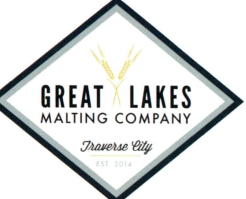

3025 Cass Road
Traverse City
greatlakesmalting.com

We believe in the power of local.

Great Lakes Malting Company, located in Traverse City, MI, produces an assortment of malted grains for the brewing and distilling industries. Our mission is to supply the highest quality malt while providing unparalleled service and an unwavering commitment to supporting local agriculture.

Michigan is already recognized as "The Great Beer State". By promoting our region's agricultural capabilities, and in turn, producing high quality, locally sourced malted grains, that reputation can only grow stronger. Great Lakes Malting believes in the power of local. Our local agriculture, our local community and our local beer!

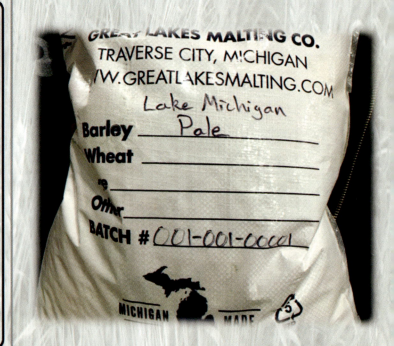

Great Lakes Malting Co. – Jeff Malkiewicz

President and Co-Founder: Jeff Malkiewicz

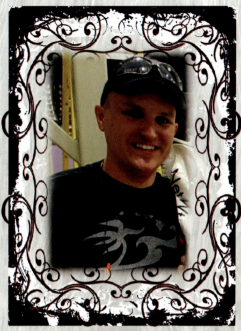

Background: "My background is in finance, but I wanted to be my own boss. I'm from Michigan originally, but moved to Northern California for work. I loved the local farm-to-table food scene there and after moving back home to Michigan I wanted to find a way be a part of that movement. A visit and tour at Grand Traverse Distillery really got my wheels turning. At that time, they sourced all of their ingredients locally except malt. After lots of research, help from my alma mater, MSU and a class at The Canadian Malting Barley Technical Centre in Winnipeg, Great Lakes Malting was born."

What **motivates** you? "I'm a competitive person. Malting is an established and relatively easy process, but the difficult part is creating a high quality product in repeated batches. I love the challenge of crafting consistent flavor and brewing performance in our products."

How do you decide **what to grow?** "We do not grow our own grain crops. The majority of our grains are supplied by 3 to 5 Michigan farmers located around the state to spread out the weather influence. It's important to use local products for that freshness factor."

Are you **partnering with any local breweries?** "Yes, we are. To date, Earthen Ales, Rare Bird, The Filling Station and North Peak have all brewed beers using malts exclusively from Great Lakes Malting Co."

What were your original goals and have they changed? "My ultimate aspiration is to have every brewery in Traverse City with a tap handle that uses Great Lakes Malt and expand from there. My overriding goal, though, is always consistent quality and flavor."

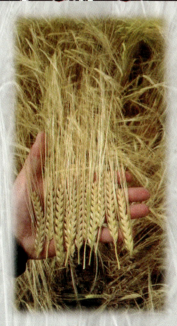

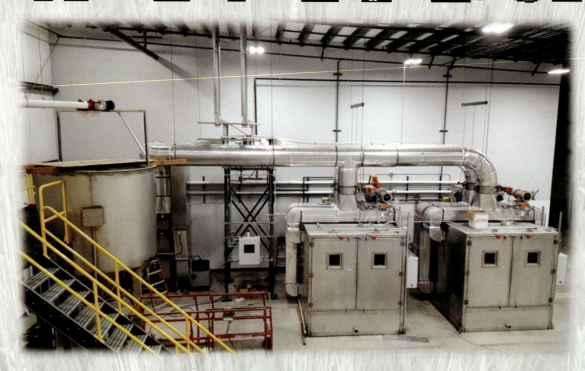
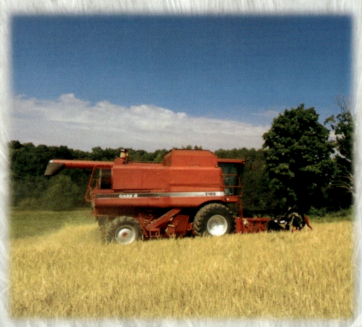
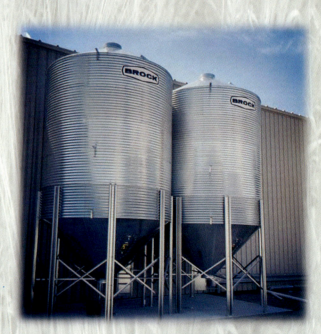

Great Lakes Malting Co. - Jeff Malkiewicz

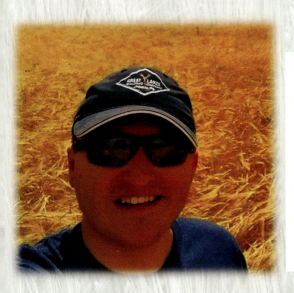

Fun fact: Jeff is an Eagle Scout. He credits scouting for helping him be prepared to be an entrepreneur and small business owner.

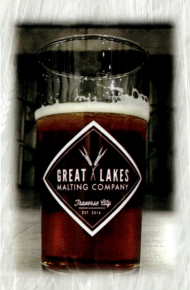

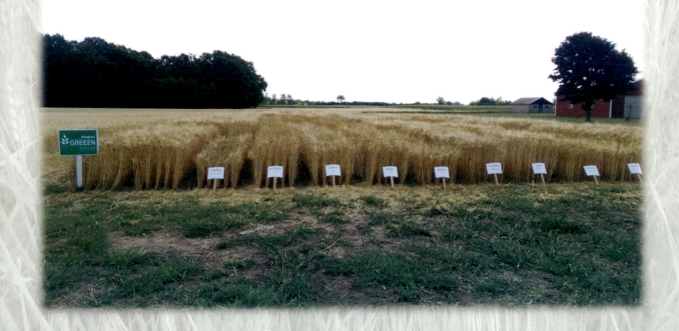

Michigan Hop Alliance

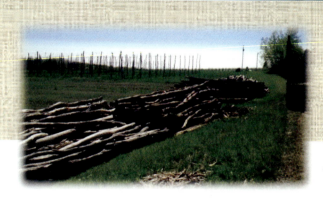

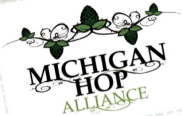

5790 Omena Point Rd.
Northport
michiganhopalliance.com

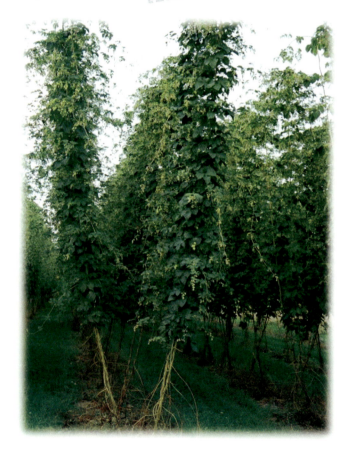

OUR MISSION

To create an environment that fosters the hop industry in Michigan through knowledge sharing and equipment availability in order to create a product for our breweries and home brewers that is superior in quality and environmental responsibility.

We are a Michigan farmer owned and sustainably grown, high quality hop producer.

Our focus is to be a resource for Michigan hop growers and to provide Michigan breweries and homebrewers with the best hops in the Midwest.

MHA can meet the needs of the most specialized breweries to the beginner homebrewing masher!

Founder / President: Brian Tennis

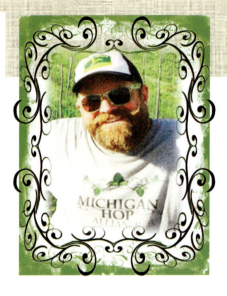

Background: "Ten years ago my wife, Amy, and I were living and working in Grand Rapids and bought a 10 acre plot in Omena for a place to camp and vacation. That land had cherry trees on it which state law requires be maintained. We tried that, but it was too difficult. We wanted to plant something else and we attended an MSU seminar about how the 45th parallel is the sweet spot for growing hops. With encouragement from Larry Mawby, one of the first grape growers on the Leelanau peninsula, we went for it and we've never looked back."

What **motivates** you? "I love what I'm doing. It's a cool industry to be in. I like coming to work and meeting all the brewers. We know some of the most important people in the industry and they are all wonderful people. Our first account was with Short's for a Harvest Ale, brewed with fresh cones. It feels good to taste what you've grown in a product you're consuming."

How do you decide **what to grow?** "Demand from the brewing community determines what we grow. Besides growing hops, we are hop brokers, importing hops from around the world (Australia, Czechoslovakia, France, New Zealand, and the UK among others). Our sales accounts number over 600 domestically as well as several international customers with sales topping the $2 million mark last year."

What is your **toughest challenge?** "Our biggest challenge is proprietary hops. We can't even get the rights to grow a number of popular hops because the growing rights are typically not available outside the Pacific Northwest. Our goal has been to try to be unique in order to differentiate ourselves. For example, we started out as organic hop farmers and from there branched out to include scarce varieties not widely grown in North America. Whatever we do, though, we like to focus on Michigan first."

What were your original goals and have they changed? "We started out screwing around with growing hops as a fun thing to do on our property. We'd always been craft beer fans so hops seemed like a good idea to try. When it came time to harvest, we discovered that hops cannot be hand picked. You need specialized, expensive equipment for picking and processing. The Michigan Hop Alliance grew from the need to purchase that equipment. We shared the equipment with other local farmers and the Hop Alliance was born."

Michigan Hop Alliance Expansion

MHA EXPANSION

StreetCar Partners, LLC has partnered with New Mission Organics and Michigan Hop Alliance. The entities will be merged and retain the name Michigan Hop Alliance under the StreetCar umbrella of companies.

The new partnership will allow for an increase in hop production—featuring even more varieties, expanded hop processing capabilities, and an expanded greenhouse operation that will supply clean hop plants for MHA and fellow hop farmers. In addition to the new partnership with StreetCar, MHA has agreed to become the exclusive distributor for the hop farming and processing group Old Mission Hop Exchange of nearby Grand Traverse County. They were also able to purchase Neptune Hops in Cedar, Michigan.

The recent acquisition of Arbor Brewing in Ann Arbor is an exciting development. The goal will be to produce beer made with 100% Michigan products.

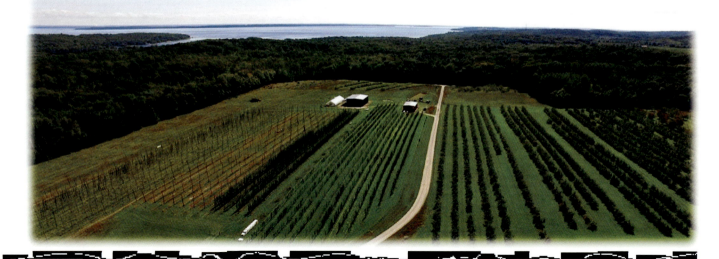

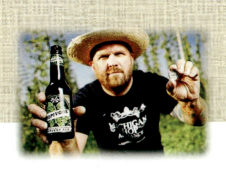

Fun fact: Brian is a former professional DJ, waiter, and record store manager – anything but a farmer!

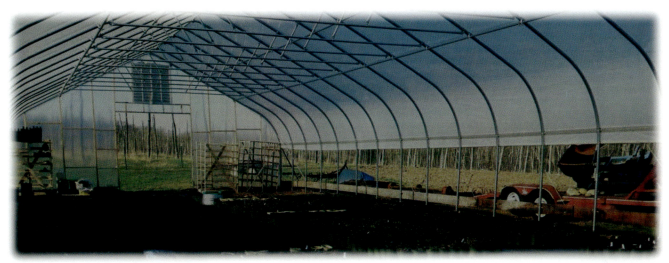

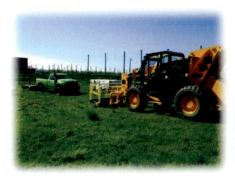
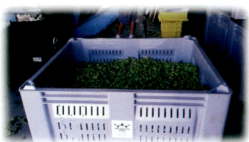
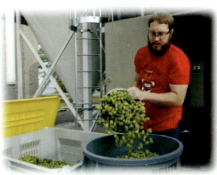

Paddle for Pints, Kayak, Bike and Brew and TC Brew Bus / Owner: Troy Daily

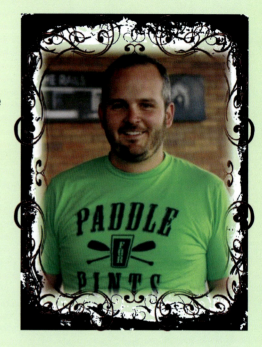

Background: "I am a native Traverse City resident who grew up in a fudge family. My family owns Kilwins downtown. After graduating from Michigan State with my hospitality degree I moved to Williamsburg, Virginia and opened a Kilwins. I got homesick and moved back to Traverse City in 2012. After my return, I wanted to take advantage of all the breweries that were opening and work with them to create awesome events. I started out working with the TC Cycle Pub. I've now branched out to create Paddle for Pints; Kayak, Bike and Brew and the TC Brew Bus."

What **motivates** you? "I love to see people enjoying themselves. Everything we do is entertainment and I like that people choose to join in for a good time and to meet others."

What were your original goals and have they changed?
"Yes indeed. It's gotten way bigger than I imagined. My original goals were to be involved with an industry I enjoyed and to have fun. I didn't want to be a brewer so I started brainstorming and here I am. I started out small and it's just continued being successful."

Fun fact: Troy estimates that he's paddled over 5,000 loaves of Kilwins fudge in the 15 years he spent working there. His favorite flavor? That would be chocolate peanut butter!

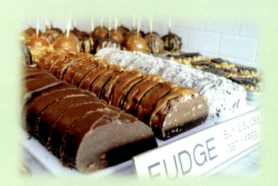

TC Brew Bus

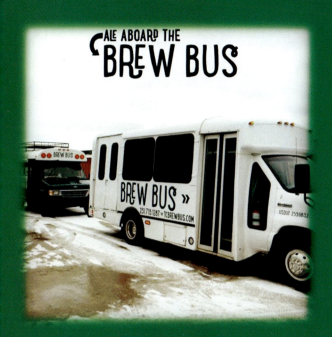

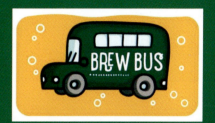

tcbrewbus.com

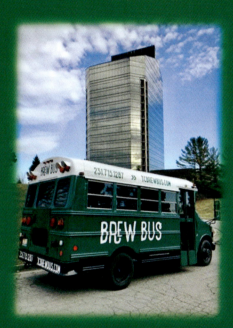

Take the **Brew Bus** for the best brewery tours in the Traverse City Area!

We do private and join-in group tours almost everyday of the week. Private tours stop at any brewery that you desire. There are over 10 breweries in the immediate area and each brewery is unique and has something special to offer.

If you're looking for your own private transportation, we also do weddings, event transportation, shuttle service and much more.

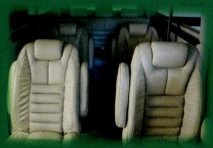

Kayak, Bike and Brew

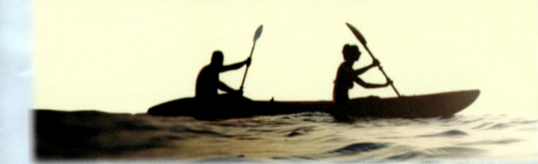

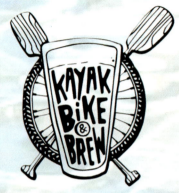

kayakbikebrew.com

Kayak, Bike & Brew is a Brewery Pub Pedal and Paddle through Traverse City's beautiful urban TART bike trails, Boardman Lake & River and West Bay, lasting about 4 hours.

Participants meet at Pangea's Pizza Pub for check-in and prepare for your bike ride. You will pedal to Right Brain Brewery where you will enjoy your first beer. Once finished we will bike to The Filling Station Microbrewery and enjoy some more delicious suds. We will launch kayaks at Hull Park directly behind The Filling Station Microbrewery.

Guides will lead you on an urban paddle through Downtown Traverse City to Rare Bird Brewpub. After completing the paddle at Clinch Park Beach we will walk back to Pangea's Pizza Pub for some refreshments on the patio. It's an adventure not to be missed!

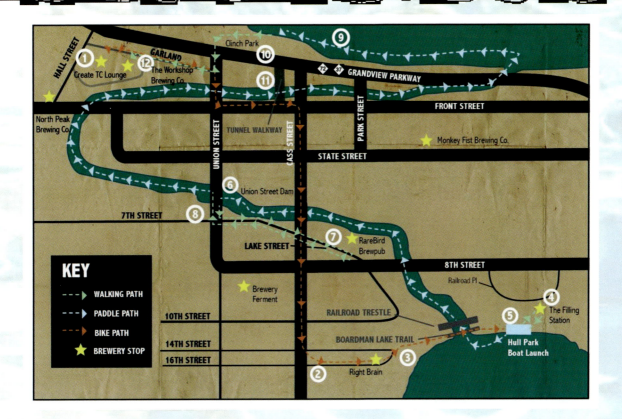

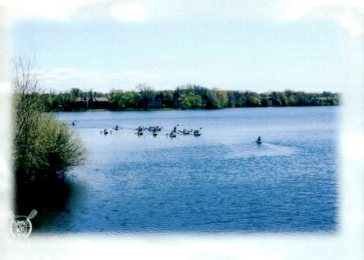
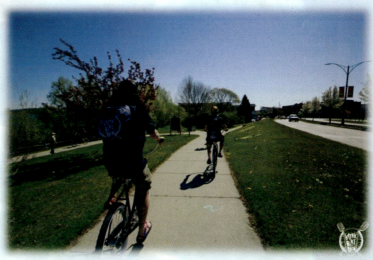

Kayak, Bike and Brew – Troy Daly

Paddle for Pints

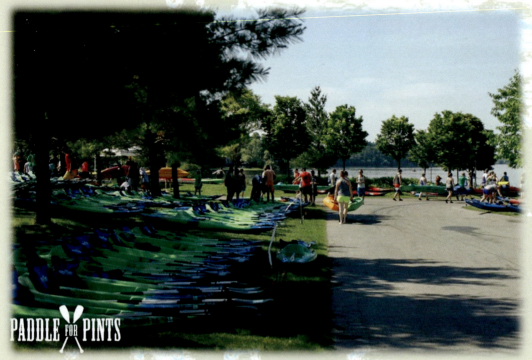

paddleforpints.com

Paddle For Pints is a brewery pub ~~crawl~~ paddle on Traverse City's beautiful Boardman Lake and River and West Bay.

Participants meet at The Filling Station Microbrewery for check-in, your first beer, and some lunch. At designated times you will launch at Hull Park directly behind the brewery.

Wave leaders guide you on an urban paddle through Downtown Traverse City over the course of 6+ hours, visiting up to 6 breweries. It's an adventure and a pub paddle not to be missed!

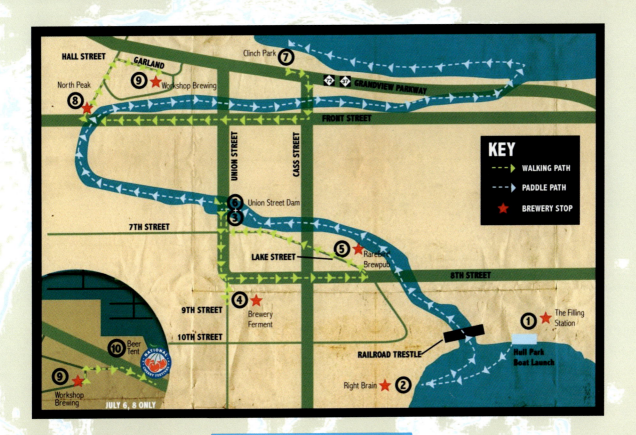

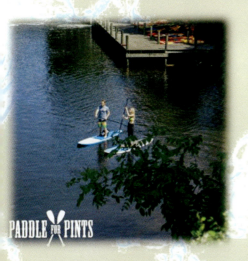

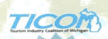

2017 **WINNER** of the first-ever Governor's Award for Innovative Tourism Collaboration in the Experience Development & Presentation category from the Tourism Industry Coalition of Michigan

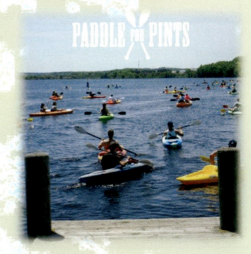

Paddle for Pints – Troy Daly

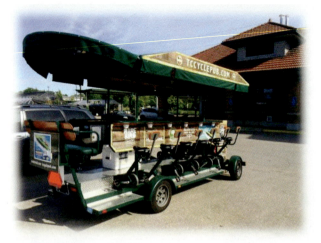

TC Cycle Pub

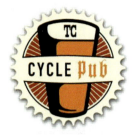

tccyclepub.com

Experience Traverse City's craft beer scene like never before! The TC Cycle Pub is a pedal-powered pub crawler built for 7-14, and the Circle Cycle seats 4-6 thirsty riders. Both bikes are powered by YOU, and driven by one of our trusty guides.

Drinking beer, wine, or cider while pedaling through beautiful downtown Traverse City, hugging Lake Michigan, and passing over the Boardman River, our 2-hour tours typically stop at 1-3 craft breweries along our route. We start and end each tour at The Filling Station Microbrewery, and our suggested stops include Rare Bird Brewery, Taproot Cider House, The Little Fleet, Olives & Wine, 7 Monks, & The Workshop Brewing Company. There are plenty of other breweries along this route as well; we're called TC Cycle Pub for a reason! Just let our friendly drivers know where you'd like to go, and we'll do our best to make it happen!

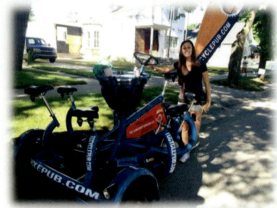

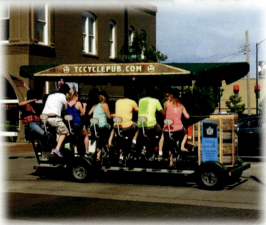

TC Cycle Pub - Kevin Farron

TC Cycle Pub / Owner: Kevin Farron

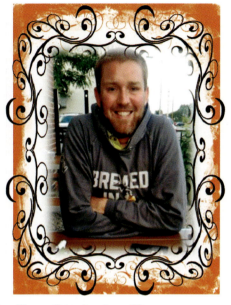

Background: "Born and raised in Traverse City, this will always be home. After graduating from the University of Michigan I moved to Bend, Oregon, where the country's first Cycle Pub popped up about eight years ago. I got to know the original Cycle Pub owner and ended up being one of the drivers. I just knew that the Cycle Pub would be a great fit for Traverse City. Five years ago my dad and I went to the city to get approval to launch the Cycle Pub. It was a challenge getting our square peg to fit in a round hole, but through persistence and many case studies to point to, we prevailed. The last hurdle was to allow drinking beer, wine, and cider on the bikes. With the help of Wayne Schmidt, state legislation was recently passed that allows drinking on board now. Every tour gets a free, unfilled growler which they are encouraged to fill at The Filling Station before we start each tour. Then riders can refill their growler at other stops along the route."

What motivates you? "It started as a fun idea to share with my hometown. Traverse City is such a beautiful place and the TC Cycle Pub adds personality to showcase the city and the beer scene in a fun, safe, and unique way. We call it a calorie neutral beer tour because you do have to pedal! As the business matures, I'm motivated to continue to improve it and ensure it stays safe. It's very satisfying when people book tours year after year to celebrate certain events. Also, when I get positive feedback or when local businesses contact me to offer discounts to our riders, it reinforces that folks really like what we're doing and the city is happy to have us. I'm all about promoting our Traverse City craft beer scene, and this is one of the best, most visible ways to do it, and the vast majority of our groups are from out of town."

What were your original goals and have they changed? "My original goal was to just get up and running, see it add to the fun and uniqueness of Traverse City, and just maybe make enough money to pay off my student loans. The Cycle Pub was built in Oregon, so the logistics of that alone presented some early challenges just getting it here. Then there was the paperwork, licensing, and insurance barriers, followed by getting beer on board approved at the state level. Now that all those original goals have been met, everything else is bonus and becoming more and more fun. I'm happy with the current state of our operation and we want to stay respectful to the town and the residents along our route, so we won't be adding more bikes."

Fun fact: Kevin unintentionally played a role in local schools' bike helmet rules and the installation of well-marked crosswalks in school zones. He had a serious bike accident as a young child riding his bike to Willow Hill elementary school. At the time, there were no helmet requirements and minimal crosswalk markings existed around schools. After the accident, all that changed. So when Kevin says that safety is a priority on the TC Cycle Pub, he means it.

Pour For More

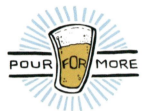

pourformore.org

Pour For More is a Michigan 5019(c)(3) non-profit organization located in Traverse City. It was established in 2016 by Rare Bird Brewpub's owner and brewer, Tina Schuett, and now consists of a board of 7 locals each contributing their own special talents.

OUR APPROACH
Micro-scale donations creating macro change in our community

Pint by pint, pour by pour: Pour For More (PFM) compounds micro-scale donations from participating vendors into a single fund that makes significant, consistent impact on local charities.

PFM participants include breweries, taprooms, wineries, coffee shops and any other establishments serving locally crafted beverages. Pour For More selects 12 Northern Michigan nonprofits annually, featuring one per month.

2017 non-profits

January- Bay Area Recycling for Charities (BARC)
February- Traverse Area District Libraries (TADL)
March- Goodwill's Food Rescue
April- Disability Network of Northern Michigan
May- Cherryland Humane Society
June- Up North Pride
July- For the Love Of Water (FLOW)
August- El Grupo Norte!
September- Child & Family Services - Third Level Crisis
October- TART Trails
November- Blackbird Arts
December- Michigan Youth Opportunities Initiative (MYOI)

Current Participating Venues

Check our website for new additions

Founder / Brewer: Tina Schuett

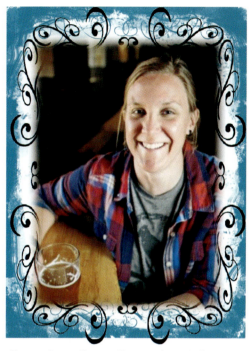

How did you come up with **the idea of Pour for More?** "I borrowed the idea from Feelgood Tap in the Detroit area with a couple of differences – we pick our charities and keep it local. Also, since we are in a seasonal business area, we don't give the donations from each month to the charity for that month. Instead, we split the funds gathered equally amongst all 12 charities. I look at this as a way for us to give back to the community without the charities having to come knocking on our doors."

Who is currently on **the board?** "Currently, we have fellow brewer Andy Largent, Chuck Pittenger (accountant), Mattias Johnson (lawyer), Marta Turnbull (media/marketing), and Troy Daly and Jeremey Smith (social footprint/events)."

How is the **money collected?** "We collect funds per pour as well as donations throughout the month. In addition, we try to do 2 or 3 events per month that feature the charity of the month and space the events out between venues. At Rare Bird, I pick one popular beer and add $1 to the price that goes directly to the Pour For More fund. Other business may choose beverage items or they might pick food items. It's up to them."

Do you have any **specific goals?** "Currently, we have 16 to 18 participating venues. I would love to get that up to 30 businesses. For the first quarter, we earned $12,000. I'm excited to see what the busy summer months bring."

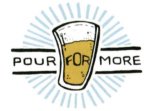

Notes

Brewpub Checklist

- ☐ Big Cat Brewing, Cedar
- ☐ Brewery Ferment, Traverse City
- ☐ Brewery Terra Firma, Traverse City
- ☐ Earthen Ales, Traverse City
- ☐ Hop Lot Brewing, Suttons Bay
- ☐ Jolly Pumpkin, Traverse City
- ☐ Lake Ann Brewing, Lake Ann
- ☐ Mackinaw Brewing, Traverse City
- ☐ North Peak, Traverse City
- ☐ Rare Bird, Traverse City
- ☐ Right Brain, Traverse City
- ☐ Seven Monks, Traverse City
- ☐ Short's, Bellaire
- ☐ Stormcloud, Frankfort
- ☐ The Filling Station, Traverse City
- ☐ The Mitten, Northport
- ☐ The Workshop, Traverse City

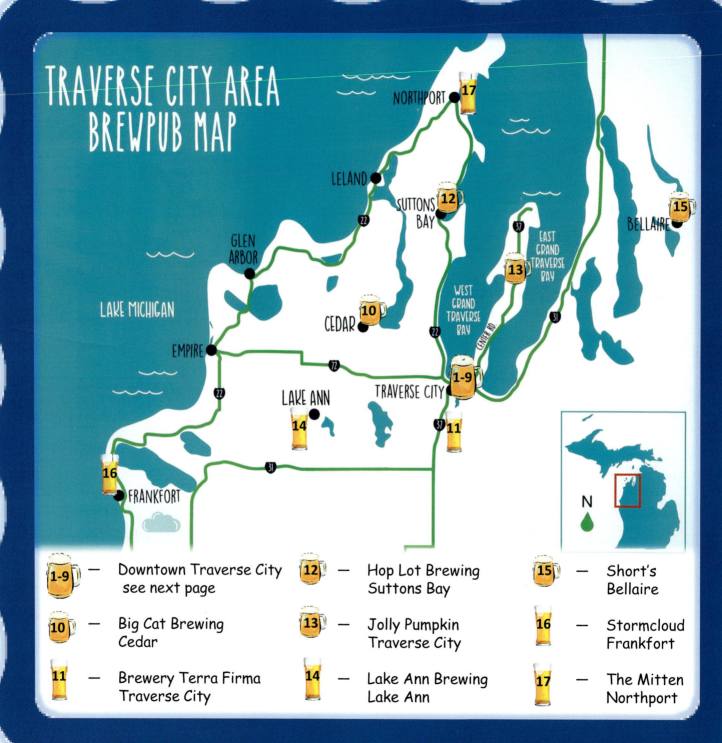

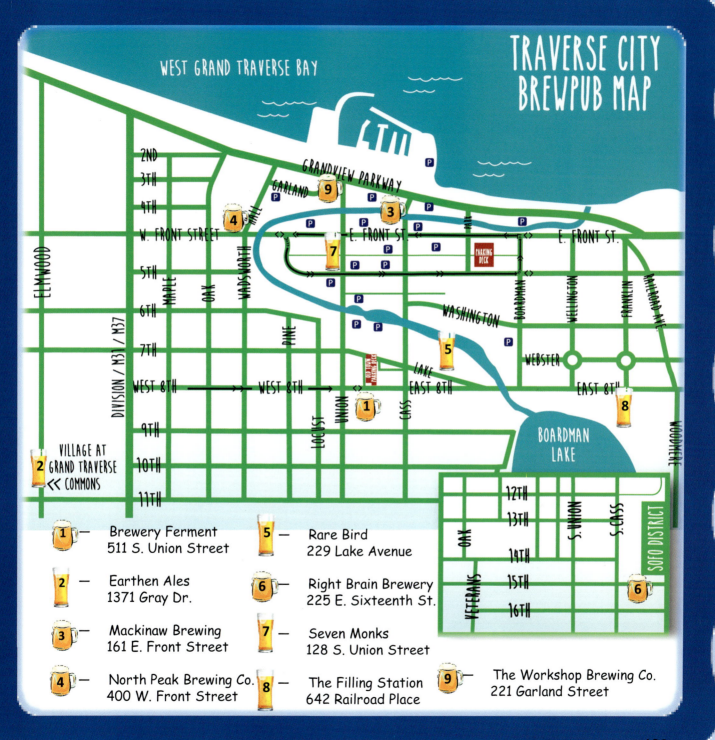

Acknowledgements

I had a blast putting this guide together. I met so many nice people and heard lots of interesting stories. Thanks to my publisher, Susan Bays, for encouraging me and helping make it all happen. Thanks to Marci Moon for help with the brewpub maps and for answering all my layout questions. Thanks to Joyce Harrington Bahle, Emmy Holman and Sandy Henschell for proofreading. And, finally, thanks to my partner, Kathy Birmingham, for her patience with this process and for always putting up with me!

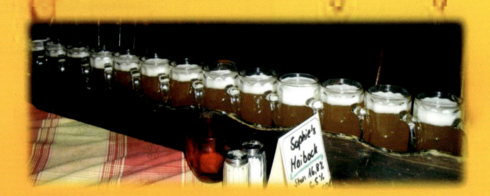